THE RENAL SLOW COOKER COOKBOOK

120+ Quick and Easy Recipes
with Low Sodium, Phosphorus, and Potassium
to Avoid Dialysis.

UMA MILLER

Introduction

The renal diet focuses primarily on supporting kidney health, because in doing so, you'll improve many other aspects of your health, as well. It can also be customized to fit all levels of kidney disease, from early stages and minor infections to more significant renal impairment and dialysis. Preventing the later stages is the primary goal, though reaching this stage can still be treated with careful consideration of your dietary choices. In addition to medical treatment, diet provides a way for you to gain control over your own health and progression. It can mean the difference between a complete renal failure or a manageable chronic condition, where you can lead a regular, enjoyable life despite having kidney issues.

Whether or not medication is a part of your treatment plan, your diet takes on a significant role in the health of your kidneys. Some herbs and vitamins can boost the medicinal properties found in foods and give your kidneys additional support, while limiting other ingredients which, in excess, can lead to complete renal failure if there are already signs of kidney impairment.

Your kidneys thrive on fresh, unprocessed foods that make it easier for your body to break down, digest, and process nutrients. Choosing natural options also eliminates or reduces the amount of sodium and refined sugars you consume, so you don't have to continuously monitor how many grams of salt or sugar are in your foods.

If you have limited access to fresh fruits or vegetables, choose frozen as the next best option, as they will have retained all or most of the nutrients in their original state. Canned vegetables and fruits are often processed, though these can be added when no other options are available. To reduce the amount of sodium they contain, rinse canned vegetables in water at least twice before adding them to your meal or dish. Canned fruit is often preserved in a thick or sugary syrup, which should be drained and rinsed before serving, to reduce the sugar content. Always read the ingredients of package or can before you consider adding it to your grocery cart, and only choose these options where fresh or frozen selections are unavailable.

Unless directed by a physician or medical specialist, don't reduce or stop taking medication for your kidneys, even if there are significant improvements to your health as a result of dietary changes and medical improvements, and there is an increase in kidney function noted. While diet should be a central part of your lifestyle, keep the medication as part of this treatment goal just the same. Any sudden or significant changes in your treatment plan can thwart any progress made, and may cause further damage in the long term. Consider your food and meal choices in the renal diet as part of a whole, which also includes exercise, medical treatment(s), and living well.

So, if you are worried that you or someone you care about may have developed kidney disease, then see your doctor right away, they will be able to run the necessary test to either confirm or deny whether you have the condition. Usually, both kidneys will be affected by the disease. As the kidneys become damaged, they will be unable to properly filter your blood, resulting in excess fluid and waste within your body. While there are often no symptoms present until the late stages of the disease, it is possible to experience side effects.

And, of course, you should be more careful of kidney disease if there is any history of it in your family. If you are prone to developing the disease, ask your doctor about a plan to monitor your kidney health in the future to prevent any damage going unchecked.

One way to go about protecting the health of your kidney is eating the right set of foods. Being conscious of what you consume. Take extra effort into knowing the science behind the food and what nutrition we get into a meal. Adapt a right attitude in your meal plans and ensure that the food you and your loved ones eat are not only delicious but healthy. Our health depends on our hands and the decisions we make even in the kitchens. Don't underestimate the value and consequences of a healthy diet.

Chapter 1. Chronic Kidney Disease

Understanding Kidney Disease

How is our health dependent on our kidneys? That's what often comes to mind when we overlook the function of our kidneys or take them for granted. Around the clock, all the waste produced and released into your blood is removed continuously—and not only that, but the kidneys are also responsible for maintaining the fluids and water levels in the body. If you consume a lot of excess water, then the excess is released out of the body by the kidneys, and in case of dehydration, more water is retained inside. All of this can happen if the kidneys are working correctly. If not, it can lead to toxic buildup in the body, which can damage kidneys, as well as other organs, and disturb the natural metabolism.

Most people are born with a kidney on each side of the body that work simultaneously to purify the blood, and both support each other in their renal function. Even when one of the kidneys loses 40 percent of its renal function, the other kidney can hide this damage until adequately checked and tested.

This is the reason patients do not come to know about the renal disease until there is enough damage done. If any of the kidneys loses its renal function below 25 percent, it must raise the alarms, as this is highly dangerous. Individuals whose renal function decreases to only 15 percent would require an external treatment or dialysis.

Chronic kidney disease is a slow-moving disease and does not cause the patient a lot of complaints in the initial stages. The group of diseases of chronic kidney disease includes several kidney diseases, in which case the renal function decreases for several years or decades. With the help of timely diagnosis and treatment can slow down and even stop the progression of kidney disease.

In international studies of renal function in many people, it was found that almost every tenth kidney was found to have impaired kidney function to one degree or another.

The three most common causes of chronic kidney disease are diabetes, high blood pressure, and glomerulonephritis.

Diabetes - in the case of this disease, various organs are damaged. With long-term diabetic kidney damage, many patients increase blood pressure and need to be treated accordingly.

High blood pressure (hypertension, primary arterial hypertension) - during hypertension, blood pressure cannot be controlled, and it begins to exceed the limits of the norm (more than 140/90 mm Hg). If this condition is permanent, it can cause chronic kidney disease, brain stroke, or myocardial infarction.

Glomerulonephritis is a disease that occurs as a result of a breakdown in the immune system, during which the filtration function of the kidneys disrupts immune inflammation. The disease can affect only the kidneys and can spread to the entire body (vacuities, lupus nephritis). Glomerulonephritis is often accompanied by high blood pressure.

Many other conditions can cause chronic kidney disease, for example: Hereditary diseases - such as, for example, polycystic kidney disease, due to which over the years a large number of cysts appear in the kidneys, which damage the functioning renal tissue and therefore develop renal failure.

Other hereditary diseases of the kidneys are much less common (Alport syndrome, Fabry disease, etc.) problems caused by obstructions in the kidneys and urine excretion - such as congenital malformations of the ureter, kidney stones, tumors or enlargement of the prostate gland in men repeated urinary tract infections or pyelonephritis.

Diagnose with Chronic Kidney Disease

To diagnose kidney disease, there are two simple tests that your family doctor can prescribe.

Blood test: glomerular filtration rate (GFR) and serum creatinine level. Creatinine is one of those end products of protein metabolism, the level of which in the blood depends on age, gender, muscle mass, nutrition, physical activity, on which foods before taking the sample (for example, a lot of meat was eaten), and some drugs. Creatinine is excreted from the body through the kidneys, and if the work of the kidneys slows down, creatinine increases.

Determining the level of creatinine alone is not sufficient for the diagnosis of chronic kidney disease since its value begins to exceed the upper limit of the norm only when GFRdecreased by half.

Urine analysis: the content of albumin in the urine is determined; also, the values of albumin and creatinine in the urine are determined by each other. Albumin is a protein in the urine that usually enters the urine in minimal quantities. Even a small increase in the level of albumin in the urine in some people may be an early sign of incipient kidney disease, especially in those with diabetes and high blood pressure. In the case of normal kidney function, albumin in the urine should be no more than 3 mg/mmol (or 30 mg g). If albumin excretion increases even more, then it already speaks of kidney disease. If albumin excretion exceeds 300 mg g, other proteins are excreted into the urine, and this condition is called proteinuria.

If the kidney is healthy, then albumin does not enter the urine.

In the case of an injured kidney, albumin begins to enter the urine.

If, after receiving the results of the urine analysis, the doctor suspects that there is a kidney disease, then an additional urine analysis is performed for albumin. If albuminuria or proteinuria is detected again within three months, then this indicates chronic kidney disease.

Additional examinations

In kidney ultrasound examination: in the diagnosis of chronic kidney disease, it is an examination of the primary choice. Ultrasound examination allows to assess the shape of the kidneys, their size, location, as well as to determine possible changes in the kidney tissue and other abnormalities that may interfere with the normal functioning of the kidneys. Ultrasound examination of the kidneys does not require special training and has no risks for the patient.

If necessary, and if a urological disease is suspected, an ultrasound examination of the urinary tract can be prescribed (as well as a residual urine analysis), and an ultrasound examination of the prostate gland can be prescribed for men and referred to a urologist for a consultation. If necessary, and if a gynecological disease is suspected, a woman is referred for consultation to a gynecologist.

What you need to know about the examination with a contrast agent, if you have chronic kidney disease

Diagnostic examinations such as magnetic resonance imaging, computed tomography, and angiography are used to diagnose and treat various diseases and injuries.

In many cases, intravenous and intra-arterial contrast agents (containing iodine or gadolinium) are used, which makes it possible to see the organs or blood vessels under study.

What is particularly important to do before the survey pole to gain in contrast substance?

If you are scheduled for an examination with a contrast agent, then you need to determine your GFR.

Together with your doctor, you can discuss and evaluate the benefits or harm to your health. If the survey is still necessary, follow the following preparation rules:

The day before the survey and the day after the survey, drink plenty of fluids (water, tea, etc.). If you are on treatment in a hospital, then you will be injected with the necessary amount of fluid through a vein by infusion. When staying in hospital treatment after examination with a contrast agent (within 48-96 hours), it is usually prescribed to determine the level of creatinine in the blood to assess renal function. In the outpatient examination with a contrast agent, your family doctor will be able to evaluate your kidney function.

Discuss with your doctor the questions about which medications should not be taken before the examination with a contrast agent. Some drugs (antibiotics, drugs against high blood pressure, etc.) along with contrasting substances begin to act as a poison. During and after the examination, in no case should you take metformin - a cure for diabetes.

Between the two examinations with a contrast agent, at the first opportunity, sufficient time should be left for the contrast agent that was used during the first examination to leave the body. It is essential to exclude repeated examinations with a large amount of contrast material.

Chapter 2. Signs, Causes and Stages of Renal Disease

The gradual and cumulative deterioration of renal function over even many years is a severe kidney condition. Ultimately, irreversible renal disease will occur in a person. Chronic kidney disorder, often referred to as chronic renal disease, chronic kidney failure, or chronic renal failure, is much more common than people realize; once the disease is well advanced, it frequently goes unreported and undiagnosed.

It is not uncommon for individuals to know that they also have chronic renal disease only when 25 % of their renal function is regular. As kidney disease grows and the organ's role is seriously compromised, harmful amounts of waste and liquid will accumulate in the body rapidly. Treatment is meant to interrupt or slow down the disease's development and is typically achieved by monitoring its root source.

Quick Chronic Renal Disorder Details

On persistent renal failure, below are a few points. The chapter provides a more comprehensive and supporting material. Blood in the urine increased blood pressure, and exhaustion are typical signs. Diabetes and also some kidney disorders, including polycystic renal disorder, are the causes. There is no treatment for chronic renal disease, which ensures symptom relief is the objective of care. Diagnosis generally takes place after a blood examination, kidney test, or biopsy.

Symptoms

Until the latter phases, persistent renal disorder never exhibits signs, but testing is advised for those at risk. Chronicle renal disease is a sluggish yet steadily progressing condition, as compared to severe renal failure. And if one kidney fails to work, regular activities may be continued out by the other. It is not generally that signs & effects are apparent until the disorder is reasonably well progressed, and the illness has become severe; at this point, much of the harm is permanent.

It is essential that individuals at higher risk of contracting renal disease frequently get their renal functions verified. Early warning will greatly help reduce major injury to the kidney.

The common symptoms of renal disease that are most prevalent include:

- Anemia
- Blood in Urine
- Dark pee
- Decreased mental alertness

- Decreased collection of urine
- Edema-swollen hands, ankles & feet (facial if serious edema)
- Exhaustion (tiredness)
- Hypertension (High BP)
- Sleeplessness (insomnia)
- Skin problems (may become stubborn)
- Loss of appetite
- Male failure (erectile dysfunction) to get or sustain an erection
- Urination more frequently, especially at night
- Cramps in the muscles
- Twitches of the muscles
- Nausea & sickness
- Hand or mid to lower back pain
- Panting (difficulty breathing)
- In urine, protein
- Rapid body weights shift
- Mysterious headaches

Stages

GFR rate shifts will determine how advanced the renal condition is. Kidney disease phases are listed as follows in the UK, and several other countries:

Stage 1: The rate of GFR is standard. Proof of kidney disease has been found, though.
Stage 2: The rate of GFR is below 90 ml, and signs of disease have been found.
Stage 3: The rate of GFR is less than 60 ml, regardless of whether there is proof of kidney failure.
Stage 4: The rate of GRF is less than 30 ml, regardless of whether there is proof of kidney failure.
Stage 5: The rate of GFR is less than 15 ml. renal dysfunction has taken effect.

The bulk of persistent kidney disorder cases only develop past Stage 2. For severe harm to be avoided, it is necessary to detect and treat kidney disease early. An annual test which tests microalbuminuria (protein in small amounts) in urine should be performed in patients with sugar. This examination may diagnose early diabetic nephropathy (early injury related to diabetes).

Chapter 3. Treatment Options

Kidney Failure Treatment

If you are diagnosed with kidney failure, you have two treatment

You can look for a donor who might donate one of their kidneys, or you may want to opt for dialysis.

Dialysis is an expensive and recurring process that you will need to do repeatedly, depending on the condition of your kidneys.

On the other hand, transplant is mostly a one-time major expense, given that you can find a perfect match.

Despite the option you choose, thousands of people have led a healthy and normal life, even with dialysis/kidney transplant. So, even if you are a victim, don't lose all your hopes just yet.

Let me talk a little bit about dialysis.

Dialysis is a process that helps to get rid of toxin and extra fluid build-up in your body through artificial means. However, an external machine won't really be able to do everything that your kidney can do, so even with dialysis; you might face some complications in the long run.

Having explained the basic concepts, there are two types of dialysis.

Peritoneal Dialysis

This form of treatment tries to cleanse your blood by utilizing the lining of your abdominal area and cleansing solution known as "Dialysate." The best part about this dialysis is that it can easily be done at home, as long as you have a clean and private area.

Hemodialysis

This particular treatment is also known as "Hemo" and is the most common kidney failure. This form of dialysis utilizes a machine to filter and clean out your blood. You should perform this at a hospital; however, if you have the budget, it is possible to do it at home.

After dialysis is the kidney transplant.

Kidney Transplant

As the name implies, a kidney transplant is essentially surgery that gives you a healthy kidney from a donor's body. It is possible to have a kidney donated from a live body or a donor who has already died but has donated their kidney for a good cause. As mentioned above, if you can get a healthy kidney, it is possible to lead a completely normal life.

And lastly, you can try medical management.

Medical Management

Suppose you have budget issues or j want to avoid dialysis or transplant altogether. In that case, there are some medical solutions that you might look into to reduce the symptoms of kidney failure.

They won't completely reverse the effects, but they might let you stay healthy until your kidneys cannot function anymore.

If you opt for medical management, then the first thing to do is consult with your physician, as they will point you in the right direction.

They will create a care plan for you that will guide you on what you should do and what you should not do.

Secure a copy of the plan wherever you go and discuss the terms with your loved ones as well.

Most people who tend to go for medical management opt for hospice care.

The fundamental aim of hospice care is to try and decrease your pain and improve the quality of your final days before you die.

In medical management, you can expect a hospice to:

Help you by providing you with a nursing home

Help your family and friends to support you

Try to improve the quality of your life as much as possible

Try to provide medications and care to help you manage your symptoms

But keep in mind that regardless of which path you take, always discuss everything with your doctor.

Chapter 4. Slowing The Progression of Kidney Disease

Keto Acid and Low-Protein Diets

Lowering dietary protein intake can slow kidney disease progression between 35% and 50% or more in many cases. Some people may go into remission using a combination of low- or very low-protein diets and the right protein supplement.

The catch is we have to know what we are doing to get the benefits or get no benefits at all. This means we can spend thousands of dollars and waste hundreds of hours with little or no benefit, not to mention the emotional toll it takes getting one bad blood test after another, thinking you are doing the right thing. Let my wasted years and money keep you from doing the same.

Keep in mind that slowing the progression by 50% or 60% is effectively a cure for many of us, depending on age. This is no small thing. If you would proceed to kidney failure in eight to ten years normally, then increasing that number to fifteen to twenty years or more is a huge benefit. Any number of things can happen, but it's not hard to imagine this delay could be life-saving for some.

There is a science to mastering these diets and protein supplements. The devil is in the details, so pay attention.

A low- (LPD) or very low-protein (VLPD) diet can slow the progression of your disease, but you can't be on a low-protein diet without compensating for the lack of protein. Some form of protein supplement is required to make a low-protein diet nutritionally safe. Low-protein diets and a protein supplement/food are tied together and cannot be separated.

Over one hundred studies are summarized at the end of the chapter. You can review them after reading the first two sections. I wanted to list every relevant study in the past ten years on keto acids and low protein. I went a little overboard, but this was needed, in my opinion. In the U.S. and many other countries, keto acids and low-protein diets are not used, for various reasons. One of those reasons is that there is not enough proof of their effectiveness. No one can say that ever again after this expanded chapter. Over eighty positive studies are shown, and I also list the inconclusive studies or had a negative outcome to be fair. It would be wrong to cherry-pick or show only the positive studies.

Having more than eighty human studies showing the benefits of any drug, food, or supplement is fantastic when you think about it. The studies include different countries and different ecologies, spread across tens of thousands of patients. When someone (even your doctor, dietician, or nutritionist) tells you this is not proven, you can hit them over the head with over eighty studies from around the world.

A key part of making this type of dietary therapy effective is understanding how these diets and supplements affect your kidneys and overall health. Again, with understanding and education comes the power to make the best decisions possible for your health and slow your disease's progression. I know it's a lot of reading, but I believe it's important to share all of the details.

Protein Supplements, Amino Acids, and Keto Acids

Protein is something we must have to survive and thrive. Our bodies can produce all but eight of the amino acids we need to survive.

Our bodies cannot produce essential amino acids. These amino acids must be provided by diet or supplementation. One other exception to this rule is tyrosine. The body can produce the hormone tyrosine, but the hormone that tells our bodies to make tyrosine is produced by the kidneys. As kidney function declines, tyrosine production is reduced.

For this reason, people with kidney disease often take tyrosine supplements along with the eight essential amino acids. However, all past keto acid supplements have been made for stage 5 patients with GFR below fifteen for renal disease. Tyrosine is neither needed nor recommended for stage 2, 3 and most stage 4 patients. Those with earlier kidney disease stages should not supplement tyrosine due to tyrosine's production of uremic toxins.

Protein Metabolism 101

Let's learn how our bodies digest protein. Amino acids have a nitrogen component. When you consume dietary protein, your body takes the amino acid and removes the nitrogen component. This is done in the liver in many cases, but other parts of the body also contribute. This process produces urea (aka nitrogen waste) and ammonia. Healthy kidneys remove both urea and ammonia. However, in our case, we have a reduced ability to remove these waste products. This is important because both uremia and excess ammonia increase the speed of kidney disease progression.

As you have learned, urinary acid and ammonia excretion decrease as GFR decreases. Patients with the lowest acid excretion rates have an 84% increased risk of fast decline in GFR. If we cannot remove the urea and ammonia, we are driving 100 mph to kidney failure.

This is important because, to a large extent, you choose how much waste product and ammonia your body produces. If your kidneys can't do the work, you need to do it for them using your diet and supplement choices.

What Are Keto Acids?

Again, amino acids contain nitrogen, but nitrogen is not used, present, or needed in the pathways that produce energy or nutrition from most essential amino acids.

Let's say this again: Your body cannot use dietary or supplemental amino acids (like those in the store) until the nitrogen component is removed for many (but not all) amino acids.

When the nitrogen is removed, the new amino acid form is called an "alpha ketoanalogue," usually referred to as "keto acids" for short. The body uses these new forms of the original amino acid from a nutrition standpoint. The new "keto acid" is the same amino acid as before, with the nitrogen removed.

Let's keep repeating important information: Keto acids, or keto alpha analogues, are the same amino acids with the nitrogen component removed. Keto acids are ready to be used by our bodies for nutrition. You might say they are the nutritional form of amino acids. Keto acids are naturally occurring in the body.

An analogy might be removing the husk from corn. The outside husk has to be removed before we can eat the corn. After you remove them, you have a big pile of corn husks to dispose of.

The parts of amino acids that we can't use have to be removed before our bodies can use them. In our case, these extra parts have to be disposed of by our kidneys. Keto acids are like buying corn that has had the husk removed. The corn is now ready to use if the husk is removed. As long as the nitrogen component is still present, your body can't use the amino acid for nutrition.

This process of removing the nitrogen component is one of the things driving us 100 mph toward kidney failure. The buildup of ammonia, urea, and uremic toxins speeds our disease's progression and eventually kills us without dialysis.

The benefit of keto acids is they are ready for our bodies to use. Keto acids don't produce nitrogen or ammonia waste products that have to be filtered by our kidneys. Keto acids are in a form that is ready for our bodies to use without producing large amounts of urea or ammonia. Keto acids go right into our bloodstreams without putting a workload on our liver or kidneys.

All manner of protein supplements exists. There are hundreds of different options for healthy people, but only two or three exist for us. Understanding how amino acid supplements stack up against both old and new keto acid supplements is mandatory.

It's all about the nitrogen

Let's start with the nitrogen amounts in each protein supplement for people with kidney disease.

Reminder: Nitrogen intake is directly proportional to the amount of uremia and uremic toxins, and your blood urea nitrogen and creatinine levels. Lower your nitrogen intake and your blood tests will improve.

Type	Daily Nitrogen mgs
100% amino acids	1,200 to 1,500 mg
Generic 1980s calcium-based blend of amino/keto acids*	500 to 900 mg
Modern 2018 magnesium-based blend of amino/keto acids	150 to 250 mg

A pure amino acid supplement may have nine to ten times the nitrogen of a modern keto amino acid supplement, depending on dosage and exact formulation.

1980s generic formulations were an improvement over amino acids, but have a much higher nitrogen content than modern blends. The 1980s blends had very large amounts of calcium—over 1,100 mg at suggested doses. Remember the dangers of supplemental calcium and heart disease. If you take 1,000 mg of supplemental calcium or more, you've assumed that you're not getting any calcium from your diet, which is impossible. Even veggies have calcium. Many greens contain 180 to 220 mg per 3 ounces, or 100 grams. Many cheeses have 1,000 mg or more Nutrition: The idea that most of us are calcium-deficient has to be questioned for heart and kidney health. Vascular calcification is the number one killer of people with kidney disease, and supplemental calcium speeds vascular calcification. These should be avoided, when possible.

Among the reasons why I think innovation must come from us, the patients. The basic keto acid supplement formula hasn't changed in thirty years, despite an overwhelming amount of evidence regarding supplemental calcium intake and vascular calcification.

A modern up-to-date approach is needed. Modern keto/amino acid formulations benefit from nitrogen levels that are three to four times lower than older formulations, and have other big advantages, such as lower calcium, increased magnesium, lower renal acid load, lower uremic toxins, and more.

Chapter 5. How to Prevent Dialysis

Being diagnosed with CKD can be a very scary and terrifying experience at first; however, you should rest easy knowing that it is still possible to lead a very healthy and enjoyable life with CKD with proper care. Once you are diagnosed, you can take certain steps to prolong the functioning of your kidney and improve your quality of life while **delaying the need for dialysis.**

Some good health practices include:

Make sure to exercise on a daily basis

Try to avoid smoking altogether

Keep your diabetes in check

Keep your blood pressure in check

Try to stay on a job that you love doing and keep your health insurance

Always consult with the individuals who are taking care of your health, such as your doctor and follow their advice

Try not to overeat and keep your weight in check

Always try to avoid adding more salt to your diet

Try to avoid excess sugar

Try to be socially active as it will help to lighten your mood

And above all, do the things that you love and try to stay positive all the time.

Is it Possible to Work During Dialysis?

Some people often think that you have to stop working or retire from your job the moment you start taking dialysis. But that's not necessarily true.

It is very much possible to keep working even after you start dialysis. In fact, it is recommended that you try to continue working in order to stay happier and healthier.

If your company provides health insurance, then you can even keep enjoying the benefits of insurance while you work. It will help you bear the costs of your dialysis as well.

There are some types of dialysis that provide more flexible treatment options, allowing you to have more time during the day for your job.

Nocturnal (Night-Time) dialysis, either at home or hospital, is perfect for these.

However, if you do start working during your dialysis, you should understand your limits. While you are working, it is possible that you might feel a bit weak or tired.

If you are following peritoneal dialysis, then you are going to need a clean place to do all your exchanges.

Alternatively, if you are on Hemo, then it is strictly prohibited for you to lift heavy objects or put excess pressure on your vascular access arm.

Depending on your dialysis type, you must talk to your social worker/doctor to adjust your dialysis routine and talk to your employer in order to reach an agreement.

Worst case scenario, if you are unable to work, you still have some options! Various federal and private programs will help you to have a stable income while keeping your insurance for your dialysis program.

Talk to your personal social worker in order to apply for these facilities.

Allowed Foods in a Renal Diet

When it comes to the renal diet and keeping your kidneys healthy, the most important thing to keep in mind is to avoid foods that are high in:

Potassium

Phosphorus

Sodium

That being said, the following food groups are strictly prohibited during a renal diet:

Vitamin and mineral supplements

Cheese

Cream soup

Dried beans/peas

Ice cream

Milk/coconut milk

Nuts, low salt snack foods

Peanut butter

Nut butter

Nutella

But don't be alarmed! There is still a bucket load of amazing ingredients that you can use to create awesome meals. These include:

Meat and Meat Substitutes

Beef

Chicken

Fish

Lamb

Tuna

Turkey

Veal

Pork Chops

Tofu

Vegetables

Beets

Arugula

Celery

Chiles

Carrots

Asparagus

Bean sprouts

Chives

Coleslaw

Corn

Cucumber

Eggplants

Endive

Ginger root

Green beans

Lettuce

Onions

Parsley

Radishes

Spaghetti squash

Turnips

Vegetable, mixed

Water chestnuts

Fruits

Apricots

Grapefruit

Lime

Pears

Tangerines

Apples

Blackberries

Peaches

Pineapple

Watermelon

Cherries

Figs

Grapes

Peach Nectar

Raspberries

Plums

Apricot nectar

Cranberries

Fruit cocktail

Lemon

Pear nectar

Chapter 6. Sodium, Potassium and Phosphorous Roles in Our Body

How Can Diet Affect Symptoms of Kidney Disease?

Modifying your diet will immensely aid in helping to control your kidney disease and prevent the later stages of kidney disease. This chapter will explore the different food and nutrient groups that you should familiarize yourself with if you have kidney disease. Always ask for your doctor's advice before changing your diet.

Carbohydrates: This makes up a large portion of your diet as they're the primary source of energy for your body.

Complex and simple are the two types of carbohydrates. An example of a simple carbohydrate is fruit. Fruit is packed with the fiber, vitamins, and energy that your body needs. Examples of complex carbohydrates are grains, bread and vegetables. All these carbohydrates provide minerals and vitamins as well as energy and fiber. Carbohydrates also play a vital role in balancing blood-sugar levels.

Protein: Repairs tissue and builds muscle. Your body also uses protein to build antibodies.

These are your body's defense against disease. Animal foods are the primary sources of protein, such as milk, beef, eggs, chicken, and pork. Protein can also be found in some plants. Legumes, nuts, and soybean products are all good sources of proteins. Vegetables also contain small amounts of protein. Protein is essential for good health; however, in later stages of chronic kidney disease, your renal dietitian may have you cut back on protein intake to help reduce stress on the kidneys.

Fats: Transport vitamins K, E, D, and A to your cells. They produce the hormones testosterone and estrogen. Some fats contain fatty acids that are good for your skin. These fatty acids also make up the linings of cells in the body and help with the transmission of nerves. However, too much fat or the wrong kind of fat in your diet can cause weight gain, leading to heart disease and many other problems with your health.

There are two types of fats: unsaturated and saturated. Meat and dairy products are saturated fats. Too much of these fats can elevate your cholesterol; this cholesterol is what causes heart disease and clogged arteries. The medical authorities advised you diminish saturated fat intake. Nuts, fish, and certain oils are good sources of unsaturated fats and all help to reduce cholesterol. Trans fats will raise cholesterol levels, just like saturated fats. The FDA suggests you choose food that is low in trans fats and saturated fats. Processed foods usually contain trans fats.

Sodium, potassium, and phosphorus: These are the three main minerals balanced by the kidneys. As chronic kidney disease gets worse, some foods will need to be avoided as your kidneys are already unable to remove the excess from these minerals. Blood tests will be conducted to monitor the levels of these minerals.

Sodium: In the early stages of kidney disease, a low sodium diet may be all you need if you have high blood pressure. Your kidneys cannot get rid of excess fluid and sodium from your body whilst experiencing kidney disease. To help identify salt in foods, look for ingredients on the label such as baking powder, sodium, or brine. Generally, children and adults should eat less than 2,300 mg of sodium a day.

Kidney disease stage 1 and 2 = 1–3.5g per day

Kidney disease stage 3 - 4 = 1–2.5g per day

Kidney disease stage 5 = 1–2g per day

Potassium: Kidneys usually get rid of excess potassium in your urine to maintain normal levels in your blood. When experiencing kidney disease, they can no longer do this effectively.

Hyperkalemia (or high potassium levels) occurs in the later stages of kidney disease. Symptoms of high potassium are a slow pulse, numbness, weakness, and nausea.

Kidney disease stage 1 and 2 = 2–5g per day

Kidney disease stage 3 - 4 =2–4g per day

Kidney disease stage 5 = 2–2.5 per day

Phosphorus: Since your kidneys can no longer remove phosphorus from your blood and urine, hyperphosphatemia or high phosphorus may become a problem during stage 4 or 5 kidney disease.

Kidney disease stage 1 and 2 = up to 1000mg per day

Kidney disease stage 3–4 (GFR of 25–90+) = p to 1000mg per day

Kidney disease stage 4 (GFR of 15–25) = up to 750mg per day

Kidney disease stage 4 (GFR of 5–15) = up to 7mg per kg of body weight

What to Eat and Avoid in the Renal Diet

As specified above, some nutrients should be limited in the renal diet, e.g., phosphorus, potassium, and thus any foods that contain high amounts of these should be taken only in low amounts and not on a daily basis. The foods that should be limited are:

Bananas

Avocadoes

Beetroots

Dried beans

Dried fruit

Mangos

Melons

Molasses

Nuts and seeds

Oranges

Parsnips

Spinach

Potatoes

Fish

Low-fat yogurt

Be attentive! The following foods have a high amount of sodium, and their consumption should be limited:

Salty snacks, e.g., pretzels, potato chips, packed popcorn etc.

Savory pies, e.g., cheese pies, sausage rolls, and Greek spinach pies

Processed meats, e.g., luncheon meat, salami, sausages

Pickled foods in salt brine

Condiments, e.g., ketchup, mustard, and mayo

Soy sauce

Canned soups and sauces

Now, here are the top foods you can consume without any (strict) restrictions, as they are naturally low in potassium, phosphorus, and sodium:

Cabbage

Cucumber

Broccoli

Cauliflower

Brussels sprouts

Onions

Garlic

Apples

Berries (blueberries, cranberries, berries, strawberries)

Cherries

Red grapes

Egg whites

Wild-caught fish

Olive oil

Bulgur wheat

Oatmeal

Skinless chicken and turkey

Arugula

Macadamia Nuts

Radishes

Shiitake mushrooms

Pineapple

Grapefruits

Kale

Ginger

All spices and herbs

Red meat and dairy can also be consumed in moderation, but they should not be combined with high phosphorus, potassium, or sodium foods as they contain moderate amounts of these alone.

Chapter 7. Renal Diet and Its Benefits

Since the Renal Diet is generally a Low Sodium, Low Phosphorus program, there are certain health benefits that you will enjoy from this diet. (Apart from improving your kidney health). Some of the crucial ones are as follows:

It helps to lower blood pressure

It helps to lower your LDL cholesterol

It helps to lower your risk of having a heart attack

It helps to prevent heart failure

It decreases the possibility of having a stroke

It helps to protect your vision

It helps to improve your memory

It helps to lower the possibility of dementia

It helps to build stronger bones

Common Questions about the Renal Diet

Adapting to a new diet is a journey that brings about a lot of discoveries and questions about additional changes and options. The Renal Diet is no exception, and while it can be modified to suit custom preferences and tastes, you may have questions about the choices you make and how different foods and drinks affect your kidneys' health.

Question

Is a plant-based diet required to maximize the benefits of a renal diet?

Answer

A vegan diet is not a requirement of the renal diet, though it can be a great benefit if this is your preference. The most crucial aspect of eating well is to focus on fresh, plant-based foods, as they are easy to digest and contain significant amounts of nutrients. If you choose lean meats as part of your meal plan, be sure to include as many protein and glow foods limit the portions of animal protein with each serving, while increasing the amount of fiber and other nutrients.

Question

What happens if I find out that a specific food in my diet is too high in sodium, phosphorus, potassium or protein? Do I have to eliminate it completely, or may I indulge on occasion?

Answer

If your condition is severe, you may want to consult a doctor or specialist before making a firm decision. For most people, the occasional food choice such as a banana, which is high in potassium, is not going to have a negative impact and is often offset with many other health benefits within the renal diet guidelines, if followed closely. For this reason, there should be no adverse effects on your kidneys or health overall. In some cases, a dietitian or doctor may recommend certain foods outside of the renal diet if they notice a significant improvement in your kidneys and to treat another ailment that could be related to kidney issues, such as high blood pressure or diabetes.

Question

What happens if I eat too much of the wrong foods and get off track. Is it too late to start the diet over again?

Answer

While it's important to adhere to this diet as much as possible, especially in more severe cases where renal function is low, don't get distracted with making the wrong food choices by switching back immediately. The odd "slip up" is expected, and anyone can make this error from time to time.

The crucial thins is to take note the basis of your food choices with your kidneys in mind, to avoid future errors and move towards a healthier lifestyle.

Question

Can I drink the occasional soda on the renal diet? Is it acceptable if the soda is sugar-free?

Answer

Drinking soda of any kind should be avoided, as the sugar content is so high (almost 30 grams of sugar in one can!). Artificial sweeteners in sugar-free sodas tend to be unhealthy and may cause unpleasant side effects of their own. If you really want soda, choose sparkling water with low sodium. Some of these drinks offer natural flavoring with little or no sugar, which makes them an excellent substitute.

Question

Is there a short list of foods to avoid?

Answer

Initially, when you begin this diet, it can be challenging to determine which foods are best to avoid. Unfortunately, while there is no short list, knowing which foods and types of meals to stay away from becomes easier in time.

Among the steps you can do is to avoid salty foods, which are known to be high in sodium and not a good fit for the renal diet. Foods high in protein should be limited as well, especially red meats. Plant-based sources of protein are much better for digestion, and easier on the kidneys. Foods high in phosphorus and potassium will become common once you familiarize yourself with them. In general, a better way to approach this diet is to focus on the foods you can have, as opposed to those you must limit or avoid.

Chapter 8. Breakfast Recipes

1. Green Breakfast Soup

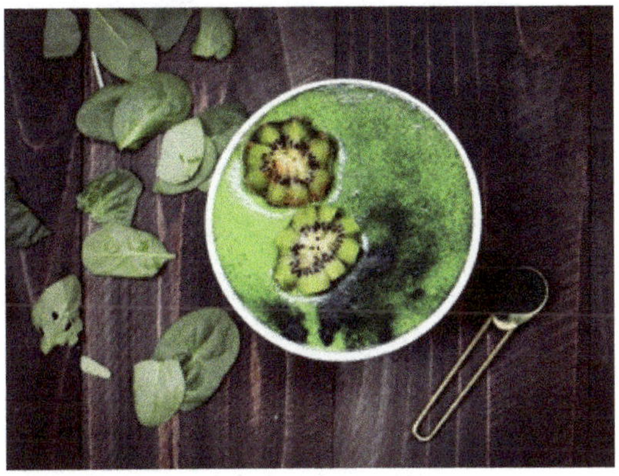

Preparation Time: 5 minutes

Cooking Time: 5 minutes

Servings: 2

Ingredients:

- 2 cups of spinach
- 1 avocado, halved
- 2 cups of low-sodium vegetable or chicken broth (lower sodium)
- 1 teaspoon of ground coriander
- 1 teaspoon of ground cumin
- 1 teaspoon of ground turmeric
- Freshly ground black pepper

Directions:

1. Using a food processor, add the spinach, avocado, broth, coriander, cumin, and turmeric. Process until smooth.
2. Transfer the mixture to a small saucepan over medium heat, and cook until heated through, 2 to 3 minutes—season with pepper.

Lower sodium tip: If you want to lower the sodium further, consider making your own Simple Chicken Broth for more control over the ingredients. Freeze the broth in 2-cup portions so you can make quick soups when needed.

Nutrition:

Calories: 221

Total Fat: 18g

Saturated Fat: 3g

Cholesterol: 0mg

Carbohydrates: 15g

Fiber: 10g

Protein: 5g

Phosphorus: 58mg

Potassium: 551mg

Sodium: 170mg

2. Peach Berry Parfait

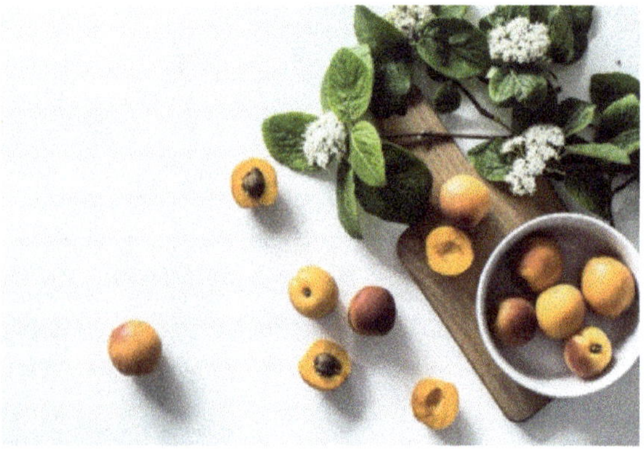

Preparation Time: 5 minutes

Cooking Time: 5 minutes

Servings: 2

Ingredients:

- 1 cup of plain, unsweetened yogurt, divided
- 1 teaspoon of vanilla extract
- 1 small peach, diced
- ½ cup of blueberries
- 2 tablespoons of walnut pieces

Directions:

1. Add the yogurt and vanilla in a bowl together, then add 2 spoonful of yogurt to each of 2 cups. Separate the diced peach and the blueberries between the cups, and top with the remaining yogurt.
2. Scatter each cup with 1 tablespoon of walnut.

Tip: Make these up to three days in advance, cover, and refrigerate until ready to eat.

Nutrition:

Calories: 191

Total Fat: 10g

Saturated Fat: 3g

Cholesterol: 15mg

Carbohydrates: 14g

Fiber: 14g

Protein: 12g

Phosphorus: 189mg

Potassium: 327mg

Sodium: 40mg

3. Open-Faced Bagel Breakfast Sandwich

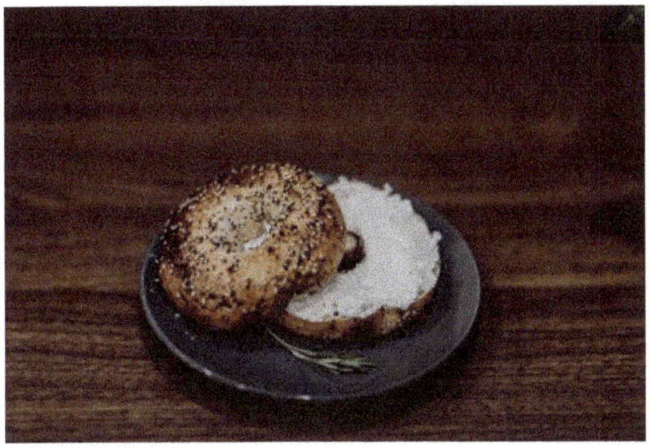

Preparation Time: 5 minutes

Cooking Time: 5 minutes

Servings: 2

Ingredients:

- 1 multigrain bagel, halved

- 2 tablespoons cream cheese, divided
- 2 slices tomato
- 1 slice red onion
- Freshly ground black pepper
- 1 cup microgreens

Directions:

1. Toast the bagel in a toaster lightly.
2. Spread the cream cheese on each of the bagel halves, then top each half with 1 slice of tomato and a couple of onion rings.
3. Season with the black pepper.
4. Top each half with ½ cup of microgreens and serve.

Nutrition:

Calories: 156

Total Fat: 6g

Saturated Fat: 3g

Cholesterol: 18mg

Carbohydrates: 22g

Fiber: 3g

Protein: 5g

Protein: 5g

Phosphorus: 98mg

Potassium: 163mg

Sodium: 195mg

4. Cauliflower Rice and Coconut

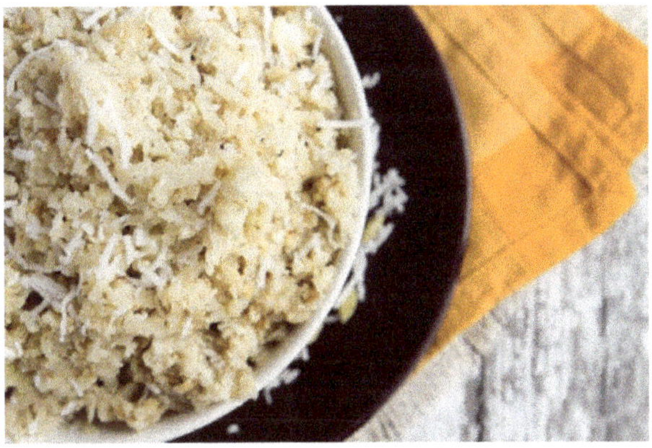

Preparation Time: 20 minutes

Cooking Time: 20 minutes

Servings: 4

Ingredients:

- 3 cups of cauliflower, riced
- 2/3 cups of full-fat coconut milk
- 1-2 teaspoons of sriracha paste
- ¼- ½ teaspoon of onion powder
- Salt as needed
- Fresh basil for garnish

Directions:

1. Take a pan and place it over medium-low heat.
2. Add all of the ingredients and stir them until fully combined.
3. Cook for about 5–10 minutes, making sure that the lid is on.
4. Remove the lid and keep cooking until there's no excess liquid.

Nutrition:

Calories: 95

Fat: 7g

Carbohydrates: 4g

Protein: 1g

5. Kale and Garlic Platter

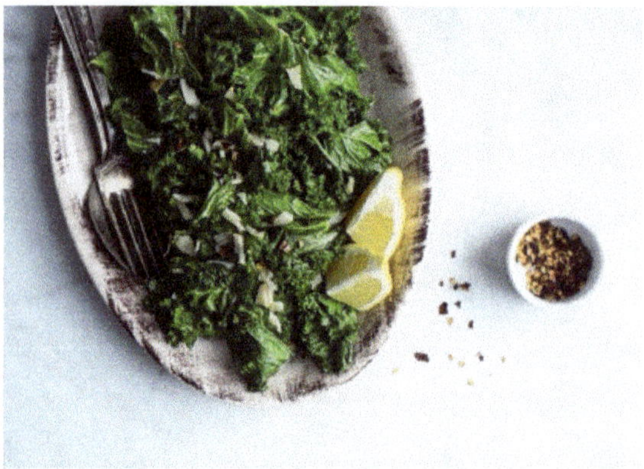

Preparation Time: 5 minutes

Cooking Time: 10 minutes

Servings: 4

Ingredients:

- 1 bunch of kale
- 2 tablespoons of olive oil
- 4 garlic cloves, minced

Directions:

1. Carefully tear the kale into bite-sized portions, making sure to remove the stem.
2. Discard the stems.
3. Add garlic and stir for 2 minutes.
4. Add kale and cook for 5–10 minutes.
5. Serve!

Nutrition:

Calories: 121

Fat: 8g

Carbohydrates: 5g

Protein: 4g

6. Blistered Beans and Almond

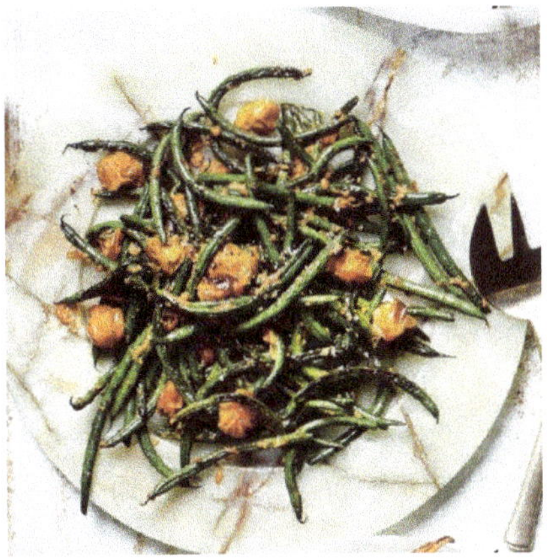

Preparation Time: 10 minutes

Cooking Time: 20 minutes

Servings: 4

Ingredients:

- 1 pound of fresh green beans with the ends trimmed
- 1 ½ tablespoon of olive oil
- ¼ teaspoon of salt
- 1 ½ tablespoon of fresh dill, minced
- Juice of 1 lemon
- ¼ cup of crushed almonds
- Salt as needed

Directions:

1. Preheat your oven to 400°F.
2. Add in the green beans with your olive oil and also the salt.
3. Then spread them in one single layer on a large-sized sheet pan.
4. Roast for 10 minutes and stir nicely, then roast for another 8–10 minutes.
5. Remove it from the oven and keep stirring in the lemon juice alongside the dill.
6. Top it with crushed almonds, some flaky sea salt and serve.

Nutrition:

Calories: 347

Fat: 16g

Carbohydrates: 6g

Protein: 45g

7. Lemon and Broccoli Platter

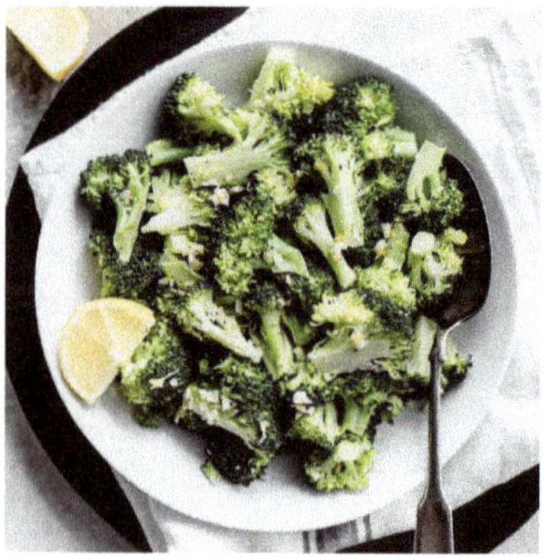

Preparation Time: 10 minutes

Cooking Time: 15 minutes

Servings: 6

Ingredients:

- 2 heads of broccoli, separated into florets
- 2 teaspoons of extra virgin olive oil
- 1 teaspoon of salt
- ½ teaspoon of black pepper
- 1 garlic clove, minced
- ½ teaspoon of lemon juice

Directions:

1. Preheat your oven to 400°F.
2. Take a large-sized bowl and add broccoli florets.
3. Drizzle olive oil and season with pepper, salt, and garlic.
4. Spread the broccoli out in a single even layer on a baking sheet.
5. Bake for 15–20 minutes until fork tender.
6. Squeeze lemon juice on top.
7. Serve and enjoy!

Nutrition:

Calories: 49

Fat: 1.9g

Carbohydrates: 7g

Protein: 3g

8. Chicken Liver Stew

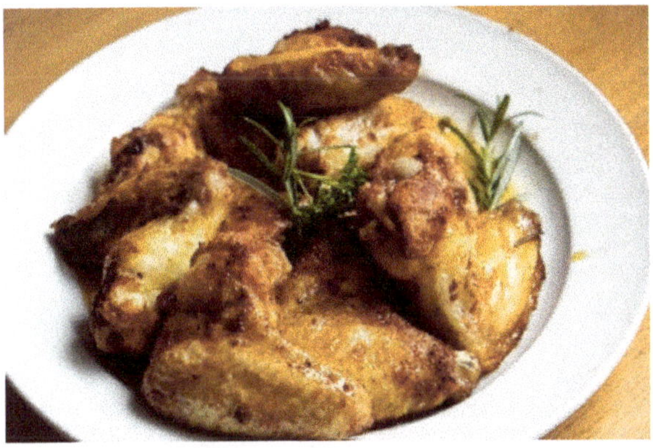

Preparation Time: 10 minutes

Cooking Time: 20 minutes

Servings: 2

Ingredients:

- 10 ounces of chicken livers
- 1 ounce of onion, chopped
- 2 ounces of sour cream
- 1 tablespoon of olive oil
- Salt to taste

Directions:

1. Take a pan and place it over medium heat.
2. Add oil and let it heat up.
3. Add onions and fry until just browned.
4. Add livers and season with salt.
5. Cook until livers are half cooked.
6. Transfer the mix to a stew pot.

7. Add sour cream and cook for 20 minutes.
8. Serve and enjoy!

Nutrition:

Calories: 146

Fat: 9g

Carbohydrates: 2g

Protein: 15g

9. Garlic and Butter-Flavored Cod

Preparation Time: 5 minutes

Cooking Time: 20 minutes

Servings: 3

Ingredients:

- 3 Cod fillets, 8 ounces each
- ¾ pound of baby bok choy halved
- 1/3 cup of almond butter, thinly sliced
- 1 ½ tablespoon of garlic, minced
- Salt and pepper to taste

Directions:

1. Preheat your oven to 400°F.
2. Cut 3 sheets of aluminum foil (large enough to fit fillet).
3. Place cod fillet on each sheet and add butter and garlic on top.
4. Add bok choy, season with pepper and salt.
5. Fold packet and enclose them in pouches.
6. Arrange on the baking sheet.
7. Bake for 20 minutes.
8. Let it cool.
9. Enjoy!

Nutrition:

Calories: 355

Fat: 21g

Carbohydrates: 3g

Protein: 37g

10. Egg White and Pepper Omelet

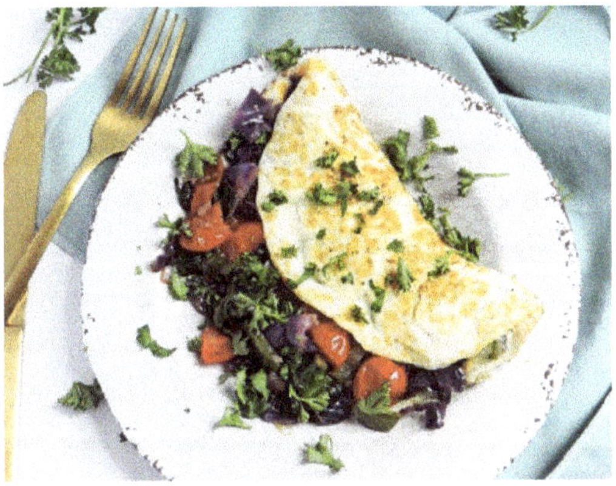

Preparation Time: 5 minutes

Cooking Time: 5 minutes

Servings: 1–2

Ingredients:

- 4 egg whites, lightly beaten
- 1 red bell pepper, diced
- 1 tsp. of paprika
- 2 tbsp. of olive oil
- ½ tsp. of salt
- Pepper

Directions:

1. In a shallow pan (around 8 inches), heat the olive oil and sauté the bell peppers until softened.
2. Add the egg whites and the paprika and fold the edges into the fluid center with a spatula and let omelet cook until eggs are fully opaque and solid—season with salt and pepper.

Nutrition:

Calories: 165

Carbohydrate: 3.8g

Protein: 9.2g

Sodium: 797mg

Potassium: 193mg

Phosphorus: 202.5mg

Dietary Fiber: 0.7g

Fat: 15.22g

Kidney Disease Stage: 2

11. Turkey Breakfast Sausage

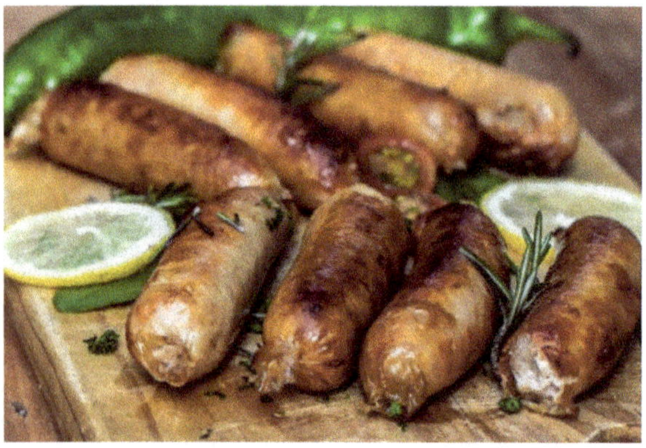

Preparation Time: 5 minutes

Cooking Time: 6 minutes

Servings: 12

Ingredients:

- (12 patties per recipe)
- 1 pound of lean ground turkey
- 1 tsp. of fennel seed
- ¼ tsp. of garlic powder
- ¼ tsp. of onion powder
- ¼ tsp. of salt
- 2 tbsp. of vegetable oil
- Pepper

Directions:

1. Combine all the ingredients apart from the vegetable oil in a mixing bowl.
2. Form into long and flat (around 4 inch-long) patties.
3. Cook 3-4 patties at a time and cook for approx. 3 minutes on each side. Repeat until you cook all patties.
4. Serve warm.

Nutrition:

Calories: 74

Carbohydrate: 0.1g

Protein: 7g

Sodium: 121.9mg

Potassium: 89.5mg

Phosphorus: 75mg

Dietary Fiber: 0g

Fat: 5.16g

Kidney Disease Stage 2

12. Italian Apple Fritters

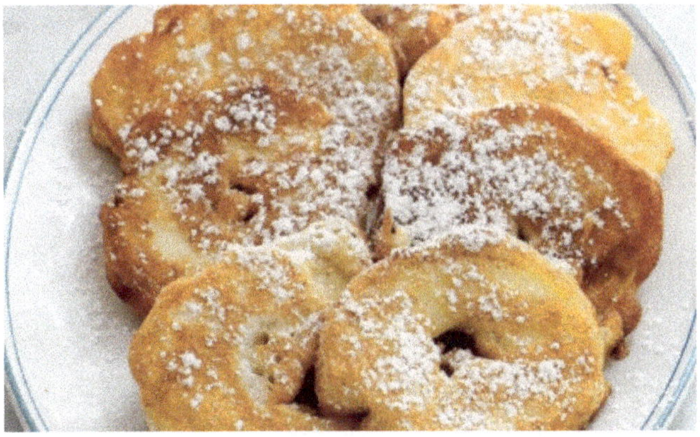

Preparation Time: 5 minutes

Cooking Time: 8 minutes

Servings: 4

Ingredients:

- 2 large apples, seeded, peeled, and thickly sliced in round circles

- 3 tbsp. of cornflour
- ½ tsp. of water
- 1 tsp. of sugar
- 1 tsp. of cinnamon
- Vegetable oil (for frying)
- Sprinkle of icing sugar or honey

Directions:

1. Combine the cornflour, water, and sugar to make your batter in a small bowl.
2. Deep the apple rounds into the cornflour mix.
3. Heat enough vegetable oil to cover half of the pan's surface over medium to high heat.
4. Add the apple rounds into the pan and cook until golden brown.
5. Transfer into a shallow dish with absorbing paper on top and sprinkle with a bit of cinnamon and icing sugar.

Nutrition:

Calories: 183

Carbohydrate: 17.9g

Protein: 0.3g

Sodium: 2g

Potassium: 100mg

Phosphorus: 12.5mg

Dietary Fiber: 1.4g

Fat: 14.17g

Kidney Disease Stage 3

13. Tofu and Mushroom Scramble

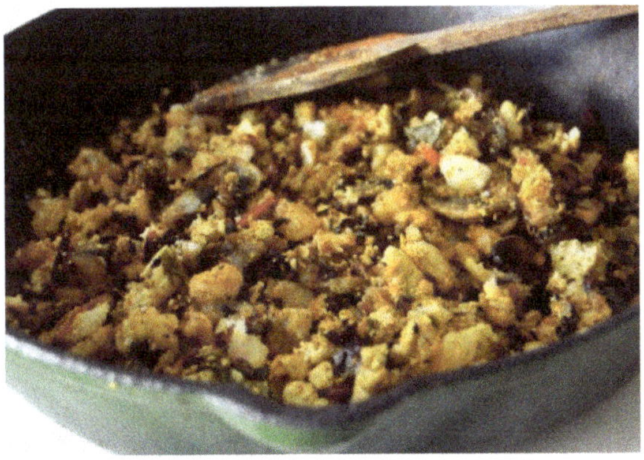

Preparation Time: 5 minutes

Cooking Time: 4 minutes

Servings: 2

Ingredients:

- Half of sliced white mushrooms
- 1/3 cup of medium-firm tofu, crumbled
- 1 tbsp. of chopped shallots
- 1/3 teaspoon of turmeric
- 1 tsp. of cumin
- 1/3 teaspoon ofsmoked paprika
- ½ tsp. of garlic salt
- Pepper
- 3 tbsp. of vegetable oil

Directions:

1. Heat the oil frying pan, set it on a medium, and saute the sliced mushrooms with the shallots until softened (around 3–4 minutes) over medium to high heat.
2. Add the tofu pieces and toss in the spices and the garlic salt. Toss lightly until tofu and mushrooms are nicely combined together.
3. Serve warm.

Nutrition:

Calories: 220

Carbohydrate: 2.59g

Protein: 3.2g

Sodium: 288 mg

Potassium: 133.5mg

Phosphorus: 68.5mg

Dietary Fiber: 1.7g

Fat: 23.7g

Kidney Disease Stage 3

14. Egg Fried Rice

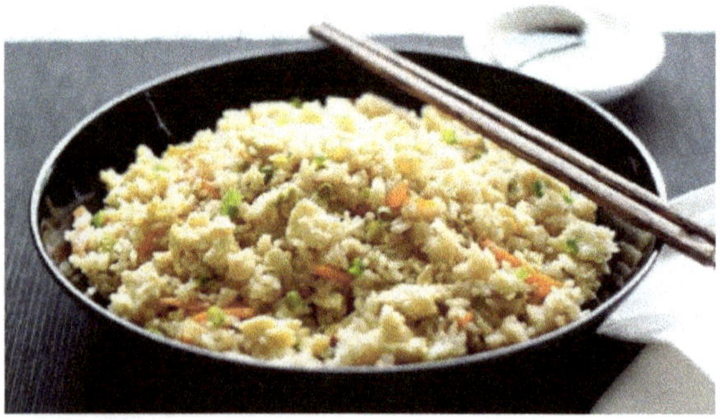

Preparation Time: 10 minutes

Cooking Time: 20 minutes

Servings: 6

Ingredients:

- 1 tablespoon of olive oil
- 1 tablespoon of grated peeled fresh ginger
- 1 teaspoon of minced garlic
- 1 cup of chopped carrots
- 1 scallion, white and green parts, chopped
- 2 tablespoons of chopped fresh cilantro
- 4 cups of cooked rice
- 1 tablespoon of low-sodium soy sauce
- 4 eggs, beaten

Directions:

1. Cook the olive oil.
2. Add the ginger and garlic, and sauté until softened, about 3 minutes.
3. Add the carrots, scallion, and cilantro, and sauté until tender, about 5 minutes.
4. Mix in the rice and soy sauce, then auté until the rice is heated through about 5 minutes.
5. Transfer the rice over to one side of the skillet, and pour the eggs into the empty space.
6. Break the eggs into a bowl and mix them into the rice.
7. Serve hot.

Low-sodium tip: Soy sauces, even low-sodium versions, are very salty. If you have extra time to spare, making your own substitution sauce is simple and effective, even if it does not taste quite the same. There are many versions of this diet-friendly sauce online, with ingredients like vinegar, molasses, garlic, and herbs.

Nutrition:

Calories: 204

Total fat: 6g

Saturated fat: 1g

Cholesterol: 141mg

Sodium: 223mg

Carbohydrates: 29g

Fiber: 1g

Phosphorus: 120mg

Protein: 8g

Kidney Disease Stage 5

15. Cottage Cheese Pancakes

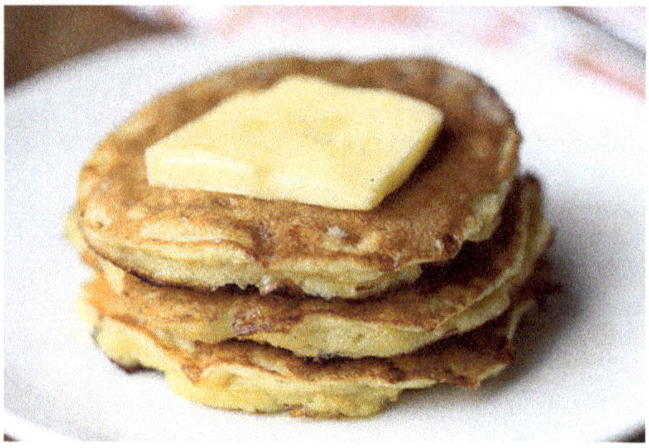

Preparation Time: 10 minutes

Cooking Time: 10

Servings: 4 minute

Ingredients:

- 1 cup of cottage cheese
- 1/3 cup of all-purpose flour
- 2 tablespoons of vegetable oil
- 3 eggs, lightly beaten

Directions:

1. Begin by beating the eggs in a suitable bowl then stir in the cottage cheese.
2. Once it is well mixed, stir in the flour.
3. Pour a teaspoon of vegetable oil in a non-stick griddle and heat it.
4. Add ¼ cup of the batter in the griddle and cook for 2 minutes per side until brown.
5. Cook more of the pancakes using the remaining batter.
6. Serve.

Nutrition:

Calories: 196

Total Fat: 11.3g

Saturated Fat: 3.1g

Cholesterol: 127mg

Sodium: 276mg

Carbohydrate: 10.3g

Dietary Fiber: 0.3g

Sugars: 0.5g

Protein: 13g

Calcium: 58mg

Phosphorous: 187mg

Potassium: 110mg

Chapter 9. Smoothies and Drink Recipe

16. Distinctive Pineapple Smoothie

Preparation Time: 5 minutes

Cooking time: 0 minutes

Servings: 2

Ingredients:

- 2 peaches, peeled, pitted, and chopped
- 1 large carrot, peeled and grated
- 1-inch piece peeled fresh ginger, lightly crushed
- 3 fresh thyme sprigs
- 10 cups water

Directions:

1. Place the peaches, carrot, ginger, and thyme in a large pitcher.
2. Pour in the water and stir the mixture.
3. Place the pitcher in the refrigerator and leave to infuse, overnight if possible.
4. Serve cold.

Nutrition:

Calories: 3;

Total fat: 0g;

Saturated fat: 0g;

Cholesterol: 0g;

Sodium: 0g;

Carbohydrates: 0g;

Fiber: 0g;

Phosphorus: 0mg;

Potassium: 4mg;

Protein: 0g

17. Baby Spinach and Dill Smoothie

Preparation Time: 5 minutes

Cooking time: 3 minutes

Servings: 2

Ingredients:

- 1 cup of fresh baby spinach leaves
- 2 tbsp. of fresh dill, chopped
- 1 ½ cup of water
- ½ avocado, chopped into cubes
- 1 tbsp. chia seeds (optional)
- 2 tbsp. of natural sweetener Stevia or Erythritol (optional)

Directions:

1. Place all ingredients into a fast-speed blender. Beat until smooth and all Ingredients united well.
2. Serve and enjoy!

Nutrition:

Calories 136

Carbohydrates: 8g

Proteins: 7g

Fat: 10g

Fiber 9g

18. Papaya Mint Water

Preparation Time: 5 minutes

Cooking time: 0 minutes

Servings: 2

Ingredients:

- 1 cup fresh papaya, peeled, seeded, and diced
- 2 tablespoons chopped fresh mint leaves

- 10 cups distilled or filtered water

Directions:

1. Place the papaya and mint in a large pitcher. Pour in the water.
2. Stir, and place the pitcher in the refrigerator to infuse, overnight if possible.
3. Serve cold.

Nutrition

Calories: 2

Total fat: 0g

Saturated fat: 0g

Cholesterol: 0g

Sodium: 0g

Carbohydrates: 0g

Fiber: 0g

Phosphorus: 0mg

Potassium: 4mg

Protein: 0g

19. Blueberries and Coconut Smoothie

Preparation Time: 5 minutes

Cooking time: 3 minutes

Servings: 5

Ingredients:

- 1 cup frozen blueberries, unsweetened
- 1 cup Stevia or Erythritol sweetener
- 2 cups coconut milk (canned)
- 1 cup fresh spinach leaves
- 2 tbsp. shredded coconut (unsweetened)
- ¾cup water

Directions:

1. Place all ingredients from the list in the food processor or your strong blender.
2. Blend for 45–60 seconds or to taste.
3. Ready for drink! Serve!

Nutrition:

Calories 190

Carbohydrates: 8g

Proteins: 3g

Fat: 18g

Fiber 2g

20. Collard Greens and Cucumber Smoothie

Preparation Time: 15 minutes

Cooking time: 5 minutes

Servings: 2

Ingredients:

- 1 cup Collard greens
- A few fresh pepper mint leaves
- 1 big cucumber
- 1 lime, freshly juiced
- ½ cups avocado sliced
- 1 ½ cup water
- 1 cup crushed ice
- Optional: ¼ cup of natural sweetener Erythritol or Stevia

Directions:

1. Rinse and clean your Collard greens from any dirt.
2. Mix all ingredients in a blender.
3. Blend until all ingredients in your smoothie are combined well.
4. Pour in a glass and drink. Enjoy!

Nutrition:

Calories 123

Carbohydrates 8g

Proteins 4g

Fat 11g

Fiber 6g

21. Creamy Dandelion Greens and Celery Smoothie

Preparation Time: 10 minutes

Cooking time: 3 minutes

Servings: 2

Ingredients:

- 1 handful of raw dandelion greens
- 2 celery sticks
- 2 tbsp. chia seeds
- 1 small piece of ginger, minced
- ½ cup almond milk
- ½ cup of water
- ½ cup plain yogurt

Directions:

1. Rinse and clean dandelion leaves from any dirt; add in a high-speed blender.
2. Clean the ginger; keep only the inner part and cut into small slices; add in a food processor.
3. Put in all remaining ingredients and blend until smooth.
4. Serve and enjoy!

Nutrition:

Calories 58

Carbohydrates 5g

Proteins 3g

Fat 6g

Fiber 3g

22. Dark Turnip Greens Smoothie

Preparation Time: 10 minutes

Cooking time: 3 minutes

Servings: 2

Ingredients:

- 1 cup raw turnip greens
- 1 ½ cup almond milk
- 1 tbsp. almond butter
- ½ cup water
- ½ tsp. cocoa powder, unsweetened
- 1 tbsp. dark chocolate chips
- ¼ tsp. cinnamon
- A pinch salt
- ½ cup crushed ice

Directions:

1. Rinse and clean turnip greens from any dirt.
2. Place the turnip greens in your blender along with all other ingredients.
3. Blend it for 45–60 seconds or until done; smooth and creamy.
4. Serve with or without crushed ice.

Nutrition:

Calories 131

Carbohydrates 6g

Proteins 4g

Fat 10g

Fiber 2.5g

23. Butter Pecan and Coconut Smoothie

Preparation Time: 5 minutes

Cooking time: 2 minutes

Servings: 2

Ingredients:

- 1 cup coconut milk, canned
- 1 scoop Butter Pecan powdered creamer
- 2 cups fresh spinach leaves, chopped
- ½ banana frozen or fresh
- 2 tbsp. stevia granulated sweetener to taste
- ½ cup water
- 1 cup ice cubes crushed

Directions:

1. Place Ingredients from the list above in your high-speed blender.
2. Blend for 35–50 seconds or until all ingredients combined well.
3. Add less or more crushed ice.
4. Drink and enjoy!

Nutrition:

Calories 268

Carbohydrates: 7g

Proteins: 6g

Fat: 26g

Fiber 1.5g

24. Fresh Cucumber, Kale and Raspberry Smoothie

Preparation Time: 10 minutes

Cooking time: 3 minutes

Servings: 3

Ingredients:

- 1 ½ cups cucumber, peeled
- ½ cup raw kale leaves
- 1 ½ cups fresh raspberries
- 1 cup almond milk
- 1 cup water
- Ice cubes crushed (optional)
- 2 tbsp. natural sweetener (Stevia, Erythritol, etc.)

Directions:

1. Add the ingredients in a blender and pulse for 35 - 40 seconds.
2. Serve into chilled glasses.
3. Add more natural sweeter if you like. Enjoy!

Nutrition:

Calories 70

Carbohydrates 8g

Proteins 3g

Fat 6g

Fiber 5g

Chapter 10. Snacks and Sides Recipes

25. Cream Cheese Tarts

Preparation time: 10 minutes

Cooking Time: 10 minutes

Servings: 6

Ingredients:

- 8 ounces cream cheese
- 2 eggs
- ¾ cup sugar
- 2 teaspoons vanilla extract
- 2 dozen paper cupcake liners
- 2 dozen vanilla wafers
- 1 ½ cups apple pie filling

Directions:

1. Preheat oven to 350°F.
2. Beat cream cheese with sugar, vanilla extract, and eggs in a mixer until smooth.
3. Layer a muffin tray with muffin cups and place one vanilla wafer in each cup.
4. Divide the cream cheese mixture into the cups, then bake for 10 minutes.
5. Allow it to cool then refrigerate for 2 hours.
6. Serve.

Nutrition:

Calories: 136

Protein: 2 g

Carbohydrates: 14 g

Fat: 8 g

Cholesterol: 28 mg

Sodium: 78 mg

Potassium: 49 mg

Calcium: 18 mg

Fiber: 0.2 g

26. Orange Biscotti

Preparation time: 10 minutes

Cooking Time: 25 minutes

Servings: 8

Ingredients:

- 2 ½ cups all-purpose flour
- 2 teaspoons baking powder
- 2 teaspoons anise seed
- 1 teaspoon orange rind, grated
- ½ cup sugar
- 1 large egg
- 2 tablespoons canola oil
- 1 teaspoon orange extract

Directions:

1. Layer a cookie sheet with a parchment sheet and keep it aside.
2. Preheat oven to 350°F.
3. Whisk flour, baking powder, anise seed, orange rind, and sugar in a bowl.
4. Beat egg with orange extract and oil in a mixer until frothy.
5. Add this egg-orange mixture to the flour mixture and mix well to form a biscotti dough.
6. Make 12-inch long biscottis out of the dough and place them on the cookie sheet.
7. Bake these biscotti for 20 minutes in the preheated oven.
8. Flip all the biscotti and bake for another 5 minutes.
9. Serve.

Nutrition:

Calories: 98

Protein: 2 g

Carbohydrates: 18 g

Fat: 2 g

Cholesterol: 12 mg

Sodium: 45 mg

Potassium: 26 mg

Phosphorus: 76 mg

Calcium: 43 mg

Fiber: 0.5 g

27. Strawberry Delight

Preparation time: 10 minutes

Cooking Time: 45 minutes

Servings: 6

Ingredients:

- 1 package angel food cake mix
- 8 ounces whipped cream cheese
- ½ cup strawberry preserves
- 2 cups whipped topping

Directions:

1. Bake the cake using the cake mix as per the package's Direction.
2. Meanwhile, beat cream cheese with strawberry preserves in a mixer until smooth.
3. Fold in whipped topping and mix gently.
4. Slice the baked cake into three layers, horizontally.
5. Spread 1/3 of the cream cheese filling over one cake layer.
6. Place the second layer on top of it and spread the 1/3 cream cheese filling over this cake.
7. Lastly, place the third cake slice over it and top it with remaining cream cheese filling.
8. Refrigerate the layered cake for 4 hours.
9. Slice and serve.

Nutrition:

Calories: 278

Protein: 5 g

Carbohydrates: 42 g

Fat: 10 g

Cholesterol: 33 mg

Sodium: 367 mg

Potassium: 125 mg

Phosphorus: 155 mg

Calcium: 81 mg

Fiber: 0 g

28. Lemon Squares

Preparation time: 10 minutes

Cooking Time: 35 minutes

Servings: 12

Ingredients:

- 1 cup powdered sugar
- 1 cup all-purpose white flour
- ½ cup unsalted butter
- 1 cup granulated sugar
- ½ teaspoon baking powder
- 2 eggs, slightly beaten
- 4 tablespoons lemon juice
- 1 tablespoon unsalted butter, softened
- 1 tablespoon lemon rind, grated

Directions:

1. Start mixing ¼ cup confectioner's sugar, ½ cup butter, and flour in a bowl.
2. Spread this crust mixture in an 8-inch square pan and press it.
3. Bake this flour crust for 15 minutes at 350°F.
4. Meanwhile, prepare the filling by beating granulated sugar, 2 tablespoons lemon juice, lemon rind, eggs, and baking powder in a mixer.

5. Spread this filling in the baked crust and bake again for 20 minutes.
6. Prepare the icing meanwhile by beating 1 tablespoon butter with 2 tablespoons lemon juice and ¾ cup confectioners' sugar.
7. Once the lemon pie is baked, allow it to cool.
8. Drizzle the icing mixture on top of the lemon pie then cut it into 36 squares.
9. Serve.

Nutrition:

Calories: 146

Protein: 2 g

Carbohydrates: 22 g

Fat: 6 g

Cholesterol: 39 mg

Sodium: 45 mg

Potassium: 22 mg

Phosphorus: 32 mg

Calcium: 16 mg

Fiber: 0.2 g

29. Simple Roasted Broccoli

Preparation Time: 5 MINUTES

Cooking Time: 20 MINUTES

Servings: 6

Ingredients:

- 2 small heads broccoli, cut into florets
- 1 tablespoon extra-virgin olive oil
- 3 garlic cloves, minced

Directions:

1. Preheat the oven to 425°F.
2. Grease the broccoli with the olive oil and garlic in a bowl. Arrange in a single layer on a baking sheet.

3. Cook for 10 minutes, then flip the broccoli and roast for an additional 10 minutes. Serve.

Cooking tip: Roasted broccoli makes for great leftovers—throw them in a quick salad for added flavor and bulk. To save leftovers, refrigerate in an airtight container for three to five days.

Nutrition:

Calories: 38

Total Fat: 2g

Saturated Fat: 0g

Cholesterol: 0mg

Carbohydrates: 4g

Fiber: 1g

Protein: 1g

Phosphorus: 32mg

Potassium: 150mg

Sodium: 15mg

30. Roasted Onion Garlic Dip

Preparation Time: 15 minutes,

Cooking Time: 1 hour

Servings: 6 [¼ cup = 1 serving]

Ingredients:

- 1 large sweet onion,
- 8 garlic cloves
- 2 teaspoons olive oil
- ½ cup light sour cream
- 1 tablespoon fresh lemon juice
- 1 tablespoon chopped fresh parsley
- 1 teaspoon chopped fresh thyme
- Freshly ground black pepper

Directions:

1. Preheat the oven to 425°F.
2. Combine the onion and garlic with the olive oil in a bowl
3. Transfer the onion and garlic to a piece of aluminum foil and wrap the vegetables loosely in a packet.
4. Layer the foil in a small baking sheet and place the sheet in the oven.
5. Cook the vegetables for 50 minutes to 1 hour, or until they are very fragrant and golden.
6. Remove the foil from the oven and allow it to cool for 15 minutes.
7. In a medium bowl, stir together the sour cream, lemon juice, parsley, thyme, and black pepper.
8. Open the foil packet carefully and transfer the vegetables to a cutting board.
9. Cut the vegetables and add them to the sour cream mixture. Stir to combine.
10. Cover the dip and chill in the refrigerator for 1 hour before serving.

Nutrition:

Calories: 44

Fat: 3g

Carbohydrates: 5g

Phosphorus: 22mg

Potassium: 79mg; Sodium: 10mg; Protein: 1g

31. Baba Ghanoush

Preparation Time: 20 minutes

Cooking Time: 30 minutes

Servings: 6

Ingredients:

- 1 medium eggplant, halved and scored with a crosshatch pattern on the cut sides
- 1 tablespoon olive oil
- 1 large sweet onion, peeled and diced
- 2 garlic cloves, halved
- 1 teaspoon ground cumin
- 1 teaspoon ground coriander

- 1 tablespoon lemon juice
- Freshly ground black pepper

Directions:

1. Preheat the oven to 400°F.
2. Line 2 baking sheets with parchment paper.
3. Cover the eggplant halves with olive oil and place them, cut-side down, on 1 baking sheet.
4. Combine the onion, garlic, 1 tablespoon olive oil, cumin, and coriander in a bowl.
5. Spread the seasoned onions on the other baking sheet.
6. Place the baking sheet in the oven then roast the onions for about 20 minutes and the eggplant for 30 minutes, or until softened and browned.
7. Remove the vegetables from the oven and scrape the eggplant flesh into a bowl.
8. Place the onions and garlic to a cutting board and chop coarsely; add to the eggplant.
9. Stir in the lemon juice and pepper.
10. Serve warm or chilled.

Nutrition:

Calories: 45

Fat: 2g

Carbohydrates: 6g

Phosphorus: 23mg

Potassium: 195mg

Sodium: 3mg

Protein: 1g

32. Cheese-Herb Dip

Preparation Time: 20 minutes

Cooking Time: 25 minutes

Servings: 8 [3 tablespoons = 1 serving]

Ingredients:

- 1 cup cream cheese
- ½ cup unsweetened rice milk

- ½ scallion, green part only, finely chopped
- 1 tablespoon chopped fresh parsley
- 1 tablespoon chopped fresh basil
- 1 tablespoon freshly squeezed lemon juice
- 1 teaspoon minced garlic
- ½ teaspoon chopped fresh thyme
- ¼ teaspoon freshly ground black pepper

Directions:

1. Combinne the cream cheese, milk, scallion, parsley, basil, lemon juice, garlic, thyme, and pepper until well combined.
2. Store the sealed container in the refrigerator for up to 1 week.

Nutrition:

Calories: 108

Fat: 10g

Carbohydrates: 3g

Phosphorus: 40mg

Potassium: 52mg

Sodium: 112mg

Protein: 2g

Chapter 11. Soup Recipes

33. Red Pepper & Brie Soup

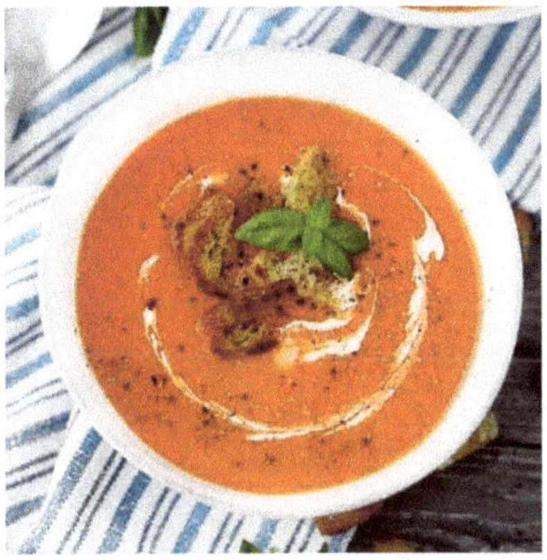

Preparation time: 10 minutes

Cooking time: 35 minutes

Servings: 4

Ingredients:

- 1 tsp. paprika
- 1 tsp. cumin
- 1 chopped red onion
- 2 chopped garlic cloves
- ¼ cup crumbled brie
- 2 tbsps. extra virgin olive oil
- 4 chopped red bell peppers
- 4 cups water.

Directions:

1. Saute the onions and peppers for 5 minutes over medium heat. Add the garlic cloves, cumin, and paprika and sauté for 3-4 minutes. Add the water and allow it to boil before turning the heat down to simmer for approximately 30 minutes.
2. Allow to cool slightly. Transfer the mixture in a food processor and blend until smooth. Pour into serving bowls and add the crumbled brie to the top with a little black pepper.
3. Enjoy!

Nutrition:

Calories: 152 Protein: 3g

Carbs: 8g Fat: 11g

Sodium: 66mg

Potassium: 270mg

Phosphorus: 207mg.

34. Turkey & Lemongrass Soup

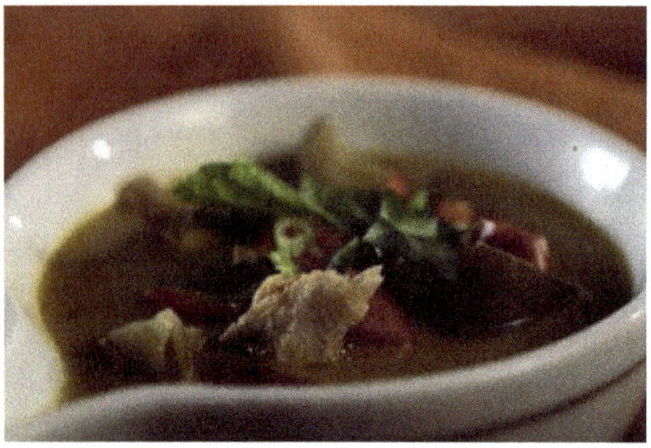

Preparation time: 5 minutes

Cooking time: 40 minutes

Servings: 4

Ingredients:

- 1 fresh lime
- ¼ cup fresh basil leaves
- 1 tbsp. cilantro
- 1 cup canned and drained water chestnuts
- 1 tbsp. coconut oil
- 1 thumb-size minced ginger piece
- 2 chopped scallions
- 1 finely chopped green chili
- 4oz. skinless and sliced turkey breasts
- 1 minced garlic clove, minced
- ½ finely sliced stick lemongrass
- 1 chopped white onion, chopped

- 4 cups water.

Directions:

1. Crush the lemongrass, cilantro, chili, 1 tbsp. oil and basil leaves using a pestle and mortar to form a paste.
2. Heat a large pan/wok with 1 tbsp. olive oil on high heat.
3. Sauté the onions, garlic, and ginger until soft.
4. Add the turkey and brown each side for 4-5 minutes.
5. Add the broth and stir.
6. Now add the paste and stir.
7. Next, add the water chestnuts, turn down the heat slightly and allow to simmer for 25-30 minutes or until turkey is thoroughly cooked through.
8. Serve hot with the green onion sprinkled over the top.

Nutrition:

Calories: 123

Protein: 10g

Carbs: 12g

Fat: 3g

Sodium: 501mg

Potassium: 151mg

Phosphorus: 110mg.

35. Paprika Pork Soup

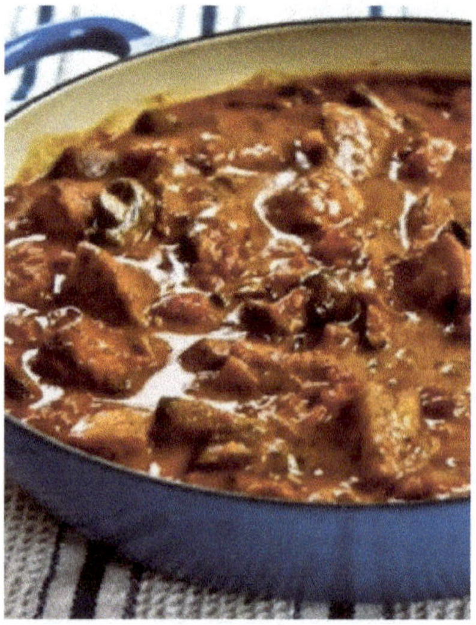

Preparation time: 10 minutes

Cooking time: 35 minutes

Servings: 4

Ingredients:

- 4 oz. sliced pork loin
- 1 tsp. black pepper
- 2 minced garlic cloves
- 1 cup baby spinach
- 3 cups water
- 1 tbsp. extra-virgin olive oil
- 1 chopped onion
- 1 tbsp. paprika.

Directions:

1. In a large pan, add the oil, chopped onion, and minced garlic.
2. Sauté for 5 minutes on low heat.
3. Add the pork slices to the onions and cook for 7-8 minutes or until browned.
4. Add the water to the pan and bring to a boil on high heat.
5. Season with pepper to serve.

Nutrition:

Calories: 165

Protein: 13g

Carbs: 10g

Fat: 9g

Sodium: 269mg

Potassium: 486mg

Phosphorus: 158mg.

36. Mediterranean Vegetable Soup

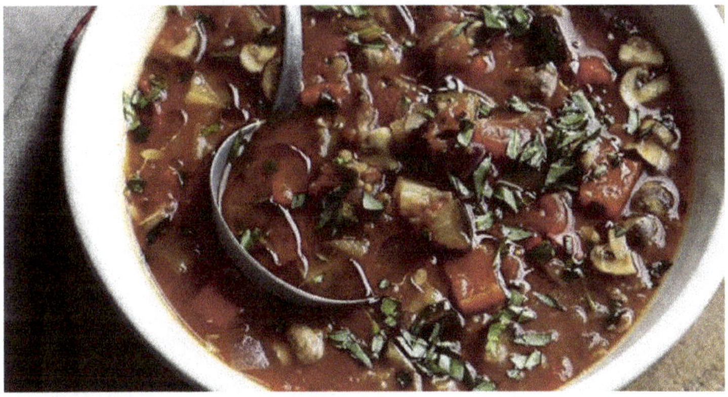

Preparation time: 5 minutes

Cooking time: 30 minutes

Servings: 4

Ingredients:

- 1 tbsp. oregano
- 2 minced garlic cloves
- 1 tsp. black pepper
- 1 diced zucchini
- 1 cup diced eggplant
- 4 cups water
- 1 diced red pepper
- 1 tbsp. extra-virgin olive oil
- 1 diced red onion.

Directions:

1. Soak the vegetables in warm water prior to use.
2. Saute chopped onion, and minced garlic.
3. Sweat for 5 minutes on low heat.
4. Add the other vegetables to the onions and cook for 7-8 minutes.
5. Add the stock to the pan and bring to a boil on high heat.
6. Stir in the herbs, reduce the heat, and simmer for a further 20 minutes or until thoroughly cooked through.
7. Season with pepper to serve.

Nutrition:

Calories: 152

Protein: 1g

Carbs: 6g

Fat: 3g

Sodium: 3mg

Potassium: 229mg

Phosphorus: 45mg.

37. Tofu Soup

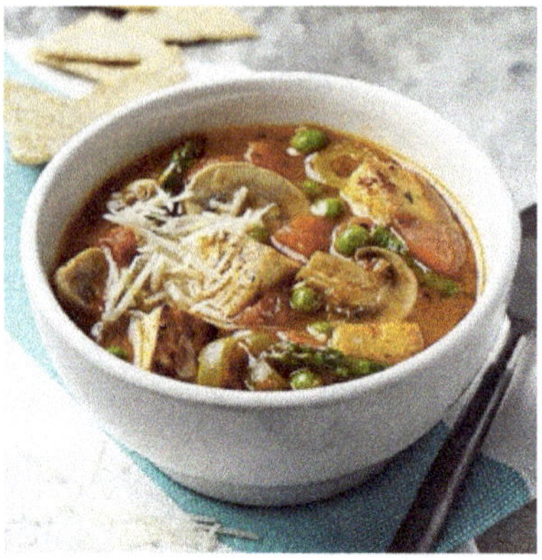

Preparation time: 5 minutes

Cooking time: 10 minutes

Servings: 2

Ingredients:

- 1 tbsp. miso paste

- 1/8 cup cubed soft tofu
- 1 chopped green onion
- ¼ cup sliced Shiitake mushrooms
- 3 cups renal stock
- 1 tbsp. soy sauce.

Directions:

1. Take a saucepan, pour the stock into this pan and let it boil on high heat. Reduce heat to medium and let this stock simmer. Add mushrooms to this stock and cook for almost 3 minutes.
2. Take a bowl and mix Soy sauce (reduced salt) and miso paste together in this bowl. Add this mixture and tofu in stock. Simmer for nearly 5 minutes and serve with chopped green onion.

Nutrition:

Calories: 129

Fat: 7.8g

Sodium: 484mg

Potassium: 435mg

Protein: 11g

Carbs: 5.5g

Phosphorus: 73.2mg.

38. Onion Soup

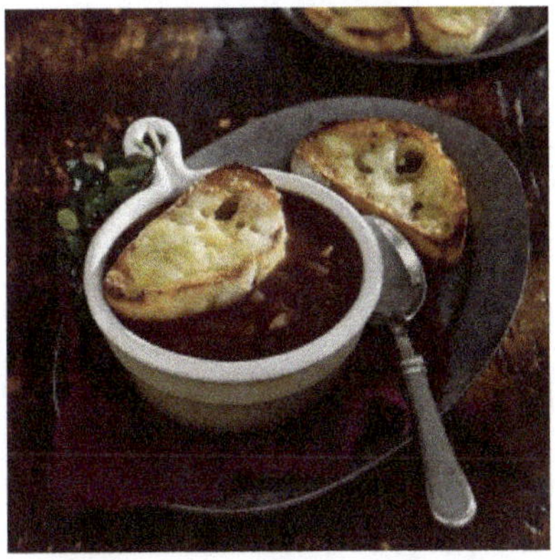

Preparation time: 15 minutes

Cooking time: 45 minutes

Servings: 6

Ingredients:

- 2 tbsps. Chicken stock
- 1 cup chopped Shiitake mushrooms
- 1 tbsp. minced chives
- 3 tsp. Beef bouillon
- 1 tsp. grated ginger root
- ½ chopped carrot
- 1 cup sliced Portobello mushrooms
- 1 chopped onion
- ½ chopped celery stalk
- 2 quarts water
- ¼ tsp. minced garlic.

Directions:

1. Take a saucepan and combine carrot, onion, celery, garlic, mushrooms (some mushrooms), and ginger in this pan.
2. Add water, beef bouillon, and chicken stock to this pan. Put this pot on high heat and let it boil.
3. Decrease flame to medium and cover this pan to cook for almost 45 minutes.
4. Put all remaining mushrooms in one separate pot.
5. Once the boiling mixture is completely done, put one strainer over this new bowl with mushrooms and strain cooked soup in this pot over mushrooms.
6. Discard solid-strained materials. Serve delicious broth with yummy mushrooms in small bowls and sprinkle chives over each bowl.

Nutrition:

Calories: 22

Fat: 0g

Sodium: 602.3mg

Potassium: 54.1mg

Carbs: 4.9g

Protein: 0.6g

Phosphorus: 15.8mg.

39. Steakhouse Soup

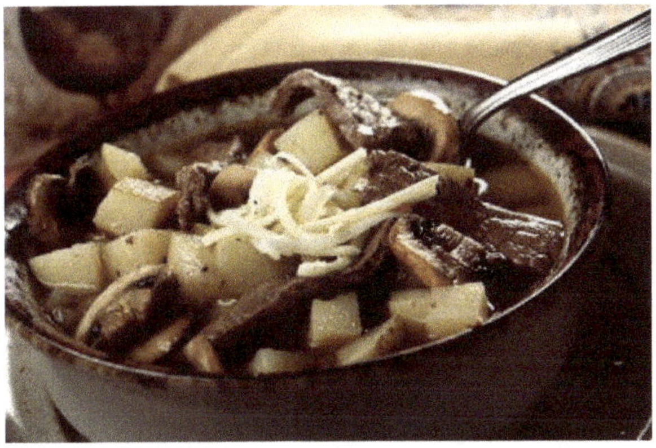

Preparation time: 15 minutes

Cooking time: 25 minutes

Servings: 4

Ingredients:

- 2 tbsps. Soy sauce
- 2 boneless and cubed chicken breasts.
- ¼ lb. halved and trimmed snow peas
- 1 tbsp. minced ginger root
- 1 minced garlic clove
- 1 cup water
- 2 chopped green onions
- 3 cups chicken stock
- 1 chopped carrot
- 3 sliced mushrooms.

Directions:

1. Take a pot and combine ginger, water, chicken stock, Soy sauce (reduced salt), and garlic in this pot.
2. Let them boil on medium heat, mix in chicken pieces, and let them simmer on low heat for almost 15 minutes to tender chicken.
3. Stir in carrot and snow peas and simmer for almost 5 minutes.
4. Add mushrooms to this blend and continue cooking to tender vegetables for nearly 3 minutes.
5. Mix in the chopped onion and serve hot.

Nutrition:

Calories: 319 Carbs: 14g

Fat: 15g

Potassium: (K) 225mg

Protein: 29g

Sodium: (Na) 389mg

Phosphorous: 190mg.

40. Pesto Green Vegetable Soup

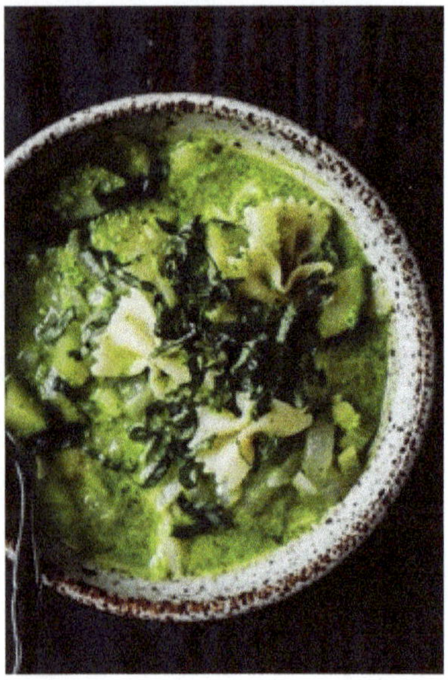

Preparation time: 10 minutes

Cooking time: 15 minutes

Servings: 6

Ingredients:

- 2 tsps of olive oil
- 1 leek, white and light green parts, sliced and washed thoroughly
- 2 celery stalks, diced
- 1 teaspoon minced garlic
- 2 cups sodium-free chicken stock
- 1 cup chopped snow peas
- 1 cup shredded spinach
- 1 tablespoon chopped fresh thyme

- Juice and zest of ½ lemon
- ¼ teaspoon freshly ground black pepper
- 1 tablespoon Basil Pesto.

Directions:

1. Heat the olive oil.
2. Add the leek, celery, and garlic, and sauté until tender, about 3 min.
3. Mix in the stock, and bring to a boil.
4. Stir in the snow peas, spinach, and thyme, and simmer for about 5 min.
5. Allow it to cool and stir in the lemon juice, lemon zest, pepper, and pesto.
6. Serve immediately.

Nutrition:

Calories: 170

Sodium: 333mg

Total Carbs: 8g

Fiber: 1g

Protein: 3g.

Chapter 12. Salad Recipes

41. Green Pea Salad

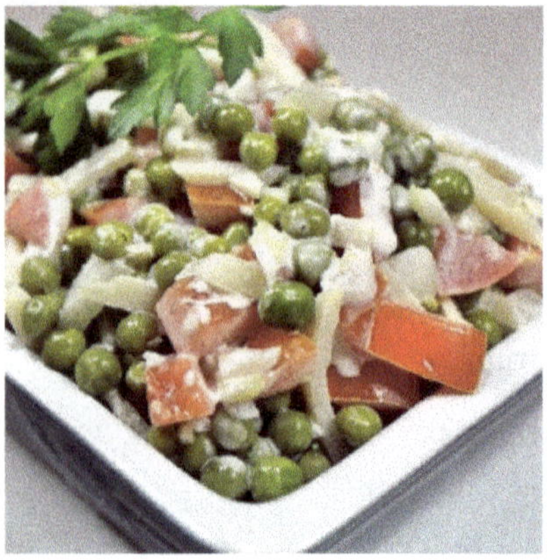

Preparation Time: 10 minutes

Cooking Time: 0 minutes

Servings: 4

Ingredients:

- ¼ cup red onion, chopped
- 2 fresh basil leaves, minced
- ¼ cup plain, low-fat Greek yogurt
- 1½ cup frozen green peas
- ¼ cup shredded mozzarella cheese
- 2 tbsp. mayonnaise

Directions:

1. Mix the yogurt and mayonnaise in a small bowl and mix well.
2. Boil the peas for 2-3 minutes, then mix the hot drained peas with the mayo mixture.
3. Add the remaining ingredients then refrigerate before serving.

Nutrition:

Calories: 132

Total Carbs: 6g

Net Carbs: 5g

Protein: 2g

Potassium: 258mg

Phosphorous: 64mg

42. Autumn Orzo Salad

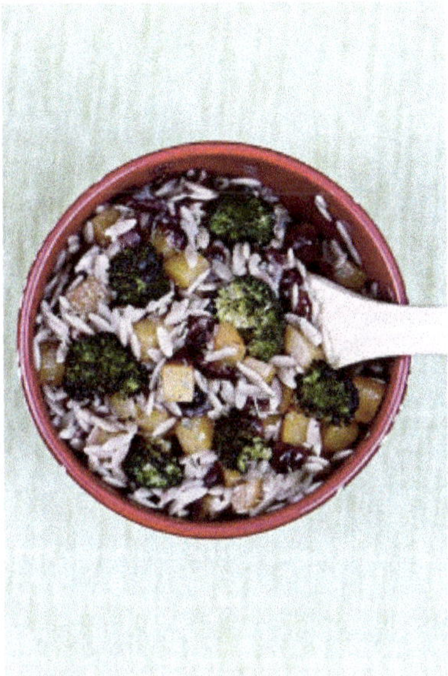

Preparation Time: 1 hour

Cooking Time: 0 minutes

Servings: 4

Ingredients

- 2 cup cooked orzo
- 1 medium apple, cored and diced
- 1 tbsp. fresh basil, chopped
- 2 tbsp. fresh lemon juice
- 2 tbsp. blanched, sliced almonds
- 2 tbsp. extra-virgin olive oil
- ¼ tsp. freshly ground black pepper

Directions

1. Combine all the ingredients except the almonds together in a large bowl.
2. Refrigerate for 3 minutes.
3. Sprinkle with the almonds when you are ready to serve.

Nutrition

Calories: 227

Total Carbs: 29g

Net Carbs: 26g

Protein: 5g

Potassium: 126mg

Phosphorous: 62mg

43. Salmon Cucumber Salad

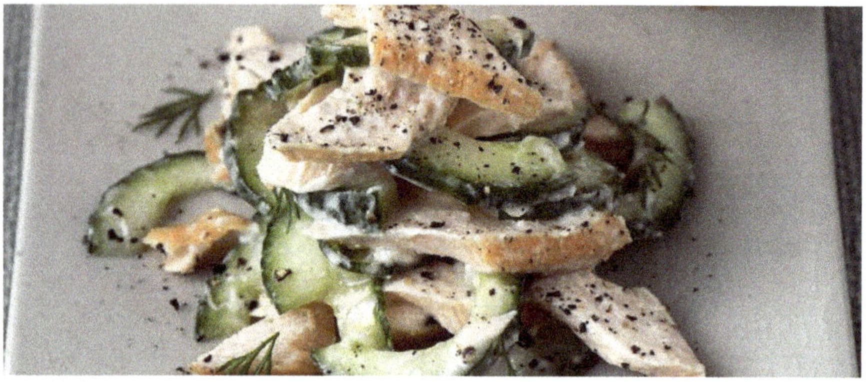

Preparation Time: 10 minutes

Cooking Time: 10 minutes

Servings: 2

Ingredients

- 1 cup diced fennel bulb
- 1 cup diced red onions
- ½ pound salmon fillets
- 1 cup cucumber, peeled and diced
- 2 tablespoons + 1 teaspoon olive oil
- 3 tablespoons apple cider vinegar
- Black pepper, to taste

Directions

1. Preheat an oven to 400 fahrenheit Oil a baking dish with 1 teaspoon olive oil.
2. Season salmon with black pepper with skin side down.

3. Placed over the baking dish, bake for 8-10 minutes until easy to flake.
4. Flake salmon and add it in a bowl.
5. In another bowl, whisk vinegar and remaining oil.
6. Add the salmon and combine it. Add remaining ingredients and combine well.
7. Serve fresh.

Nutrition

Calories: 288

Fat: 14g

Phosphorus: 217mg

Potassium: 548mg

Sodium: 178mg

Carbohydrates: 17g

Protein: 26g

44. Shrimp Mayo Salad

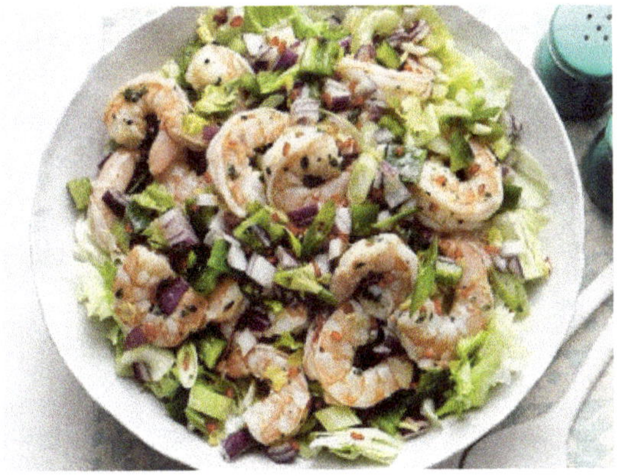

Preparation Time: 40 minutes

Cooking Time: 0 minutes

Servings: 2

Ingredients

- 1 tablespoon celery, chopped
- 1 tablespoon green pepper, chopped
- 1 tablespoon onion, chopped
- 1 pound shrimp, boiled, chopped and deveined

- 1 hard-boiled egg, chopped
- 1 teaspoon lemon juice
- 1/2 teaspoon chili powder
- 1/8 teaspoon hot sauce
- 2 tablespoons mayonnaise
- ½ teaspoon dry mustard lettuce, chopped or shredded (optional)
- Lettuce leaves

Directions

1. Combine all ingredients except lettuce in a mixing bowl. Combine to mix well with each other.
2. Refrigerate for 30 minutes.
3. Arrange lettuce leaves on a plate; add salad mixture on top.
4. Serve fresh.

Nutrition

Calories: 161 Fat: 5g

Phosphorus: 271mg

Potassium: 224mg

Sodium: 255mg Carbohydrates: 2g

Protein: 26g

45. Beet Feta Salad

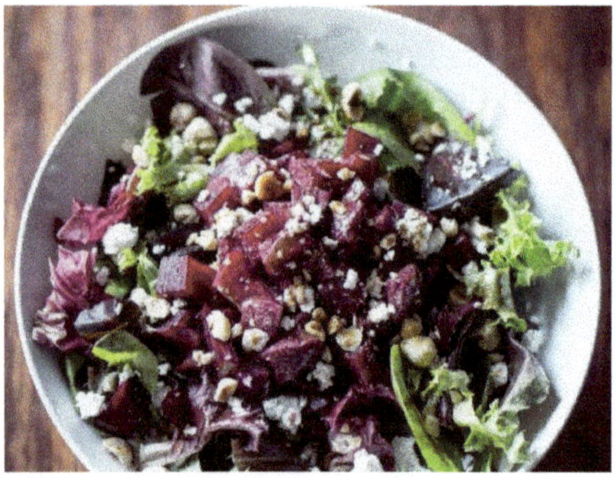

Preparation Time: 10 minutes

Cooking Time: 30 minutes

Servings: 5

Ingredients

- 4 cups baby salad greens
- ½ sweet onion, sliced
- 8 small beets, trimmed
- 2 tablespoons + 1 teaspoon extra-virgin olive oil
- 1 tablespoon white wine vinegar
- 1 teaspoon Dijon mustard
- Black pepper (ground), to taste
- 2 tablespoons crumbled feta cheese
- 2 tablespoons walnut pieces

Directions

1. Preheat an oven to 400 fahrenheit. Grease an aluminum foil with some cooking spray.
2. Add beets with 1 teaspoon of olive oil; combine and wrap foil.
3. Bake for 30 minutes until it becomes tender. Cut beets into wedges.
4. In a mixing bowl, add remaining olive oil, vinegar, black pepper, and mustard. Combine to mix well with each other.
5. In a mixing bowl, add salad greens, onion, feta cheese, and walnuts. Combine to mix well with each other.
6. Add half of the prepared vinaigrette and toss well.
7. Add beet and combine well.
8. Drizzle remaining vinaigrette and serve fresh.

Nutrition

Calories: 184 Fat: 9g

Phosphorus: 98mg

Potassium: 601mg

Sodium: 235mg Carbohydrates: 19g

Protein: 4g

46. Cabbage Pear Salad

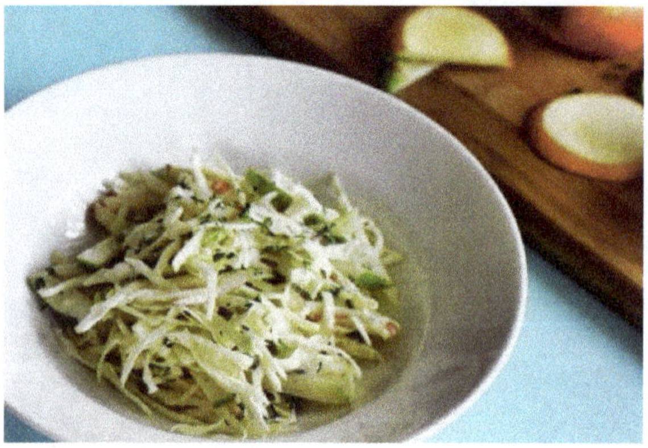

Preparation Time: 10 minutes + 1 hour

Cooking Time: 0 minutes

Servings: 6

Ingredients

- 2 scallions, chopped
- 2 cups finely shredded green cabbage
- 1 cup finely shredded red cabbage
- ½ red bell pepper, boiled and chopped
- ½ cup chopped cilantro
- 2 celery stalks, chopped
- 1 Asian pear, cored and grated
- ¼ cup olive oil
- Juice of 1 lime
- Zest of 1 lime
- 1 teaspoon granulated sugar

Directions

1. In a mixing bowl, add cabbages, scallions, celery, pear, red pepper, and cilantro. Combine to mix well with each other.
2. Take another mixing bowl; add olive oil, lime juice, lime zest, and sugar. Combine to mix well with each other.
3. Add dressing over and toss well.
4. Refrigerate for 1 hour; serve chilled.

Nutrition

Calories: 128 Fat: 8g

Phosphorus: 25mg

Potassium: 149mg

Sodium: 57mg Carbohydrates: 2g

Protein: 6g

47. Arugula Parmesan Salad

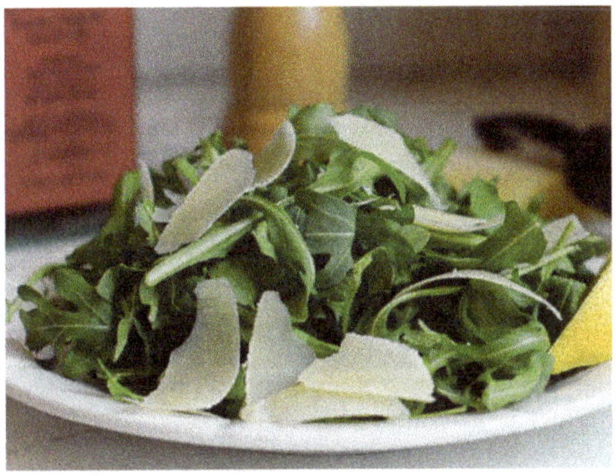

Preparation Time: 10 minutes

Cooking Time: 0 minutes

Servings: 4

Ingredients

- 2 cups loosely packed arugula
- 1 tablespoon extra-virgin olive oil
- 1 shallot, thinly sliced
- 3 celery stalks, ¼ inch thick
- 2 tablespoons white wine vinegar
- Black pepper (ground), to taste
- 2 tablespoons Parmesan cheese, grated

Directions

1. In a mixing bowl, add shallot, celery stalks, and arugula. Combine to mix well with each other.
2. Take another mixing bowl; add olive oil, vinegar, and black pepper. Combine to mix well with each other.

3. Add dressing over and toss well.
4. Add cheese on top, and serve fresh.

Nutrition

Calories: 61

Fat: 4g

Phosphorus: 34mg

Potassium: 53mg

Sodium: 55mg

Carbohydrates: 1g

Protein: 2g

48. Asian Cabbage Slaw

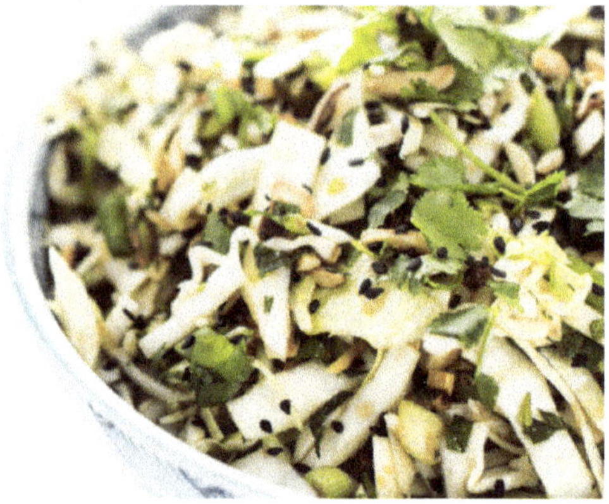

Preparation Time: 10 minutes

Cooking Time: 0 minutes

Servings: 4

Ingredients

- 4 cup shredded cabbage
- ¼ cup canned, sliced water chestnuts
- 3 green onions, finely diced
- 1 tbsp. sesame seeds
- ½ cup chow Mein noodles
- 2 tbsp. canola oil
- 2 tbsp. apple cider vinegar

- 2 tsp. sugar
- ¼ tsp. black pepper

Directions

1. Place vegetables and sesame seeds in a large bowl.
2. Dissolve sugar in vinegar in a small bowl.
3. Whisk in the oil.
4. Pout the dressing over the cabbage and mix until thoroughly combined.
5. Chill for several hours
6. You can add chow Mein noodles and toss before serving.

Nutrition

Calories: 130

Total Carbs: 8g

Net Carbs: 5g

Protein: 2g

Potassium: 183mg

Phosphorous: 50mg

49. Carrot and Lemon Salad

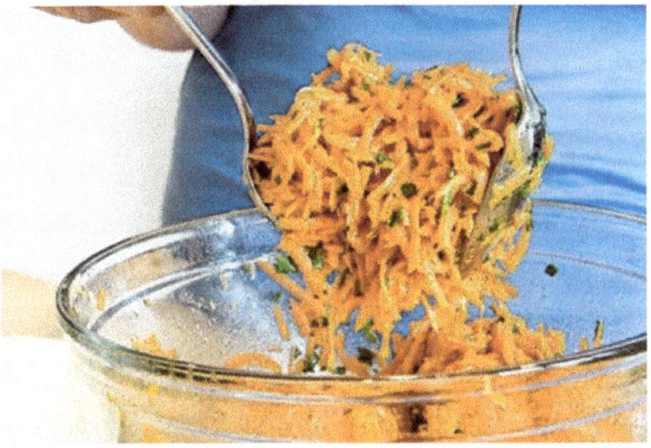

Preparation Time: 1 hour 10 minutes

Cooking Time: 0 minutes

Servings: 4

Ingredients

- 4 cup fresh carrots
- 5 lemons
- ½ cup granulated sugar

Directions

1. Shred carrots in a food processor.
2. Wash the lemons and remove the tips. Roughly chop the lemon and add to the food processor with carrots.
3. Stir in the sugar and chill in the refrigerator for one hour before serving.

Nutrition

Calories: 68

Total Carbs: 16g

Net Carbs: 12g

Protein: 1g

Potassium: 220mg

Phosphorous: 17mg

50. Heart Healthy Chicken Salad

Preparation Time: 10 minutes

Cooking Time: 60 minutes

Servings: 4

Ingredients:

- 3 tbsps mayonnaise, low-fat
- ½ tsp onion powder
- 1 tbsp lemon juice
- ¼ cup celery (chopped)
- 3 ¼ cups chicken breast (cooked, cubed, and skinless)

Directions:

1. Bake chicken breasts for 45 minutes at 350oF.Allow it to cool and cut them into cubes and place them in the refrigerator.
2. Combine all other ingredients in a large bowl then add the chilled chicken.
3. Mix well and ready to serve.
4. Enjoy!

Nutrition:

Calories: 408;

carbs: 1g;

protein: 50g;

fats: 22g;

phosphorus: 413mg;

potassium: 542mg;

sodium: 154mg

Chapter 13. Fish and Seafood Recipes

51. Shrimp Paella

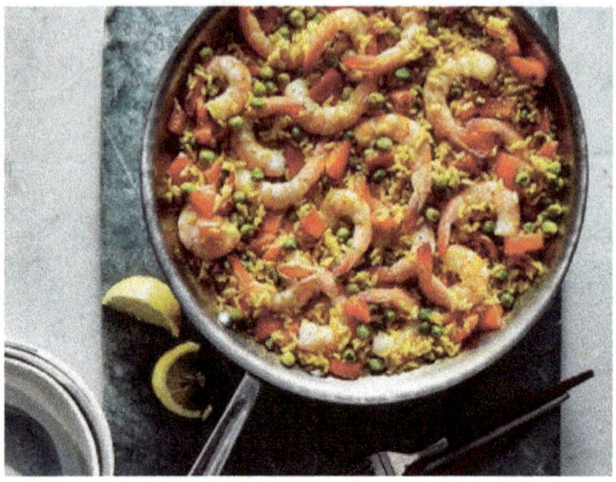

Preparation time: 5 minutes

Cooking time: 10 minutes

Servings: 2

Ingredients:

- 1 cup cooked brown rice
- 1 chopped red onion
- 1 tsp. paprika
- 1 chopped garlic clove
- 1 tbsp. olive oil
- 6 oz. frozen cooked shrimp
- 1 deseeded and sliced chili pepper
- 1 tbsp. oregano

Directions:

1. Heat the olive oil in a large pan on medium-high heat.
2. Add the onion and garlic and sauté for 2-3 minutes until soft.
3. Now add the shrimp and sauté for a further 5 minutes or until hot through.
4. Now add the herbs, spices, chili and rice with 1/2 cup boiling water.
5. Stir until everything is warm and the water has been absorbed.
6. Plate up and serve.

Nutrition:

Calories 221

Protein 17 g

Carbs 31 g

Fat 8 g

Sodium (Na) 235 mg

Potassium (K) 176 mg

Phosphorus 189 mg

52. Salmon & Pesto Salad

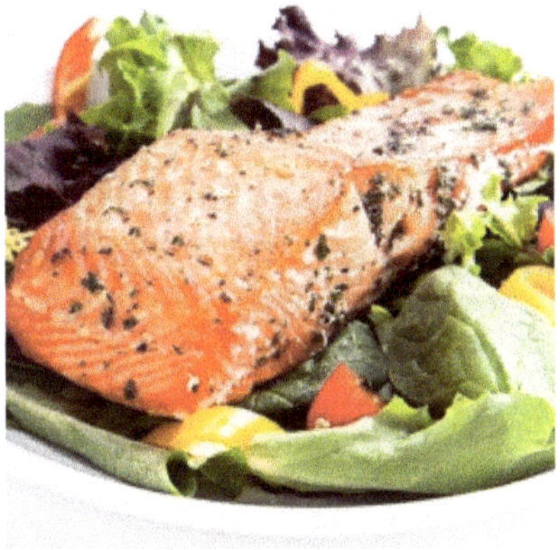

Preparation time: 5 minutes

Cooking time: 15 minutes

Servings: 2

Ingredients:

For the pesto:

- 1 minced garlic clove
- ½ cup fresh arugula
- ¼ cup extra virgin olive oi l
- ½ cup fresh basil
- 1 tsp. black pepper
- For the salmon:
- 4 oz. skinless salmon fillet
- 1 tbsp. coconut oil

For the salad:

- ½ juiced lemon
- 2 sliced radishes
- ½ cup iceberg lettuce
- 1 tsp. black pepper

Directions:

1. Prepare the pesto by blending all the ingredients for the pesto in a food processor or by grinding with a pestle and mortar. Set aside.
2. Add a skillet to the stove on medium-high heat and melt the coconut oil.
3. Add the salmon to the pan.
4. Cook for 7-8 minutes and turn over.
5. Cook for a further 3-4 minutes or until cooked through.
6. Remove fillets from the skillet and allow to rest.
7. Mix the lettuce and the radishes and squeeze over the juice of ½ lemon.
8. Flake the salmon with a fork and mix through the salad.
9. Toss to coat and sprinkle with a little black pepper to serve.

Nutrition:

Calories 221,

Protein 13 g,

Carbs 1 g,

Fat 34 g,

Sodium (Na) 80 mg,

Potassium (K) 119 mg,

Phosphorus 158 mg

53. Baked Fennel & Garlic Sea Bass

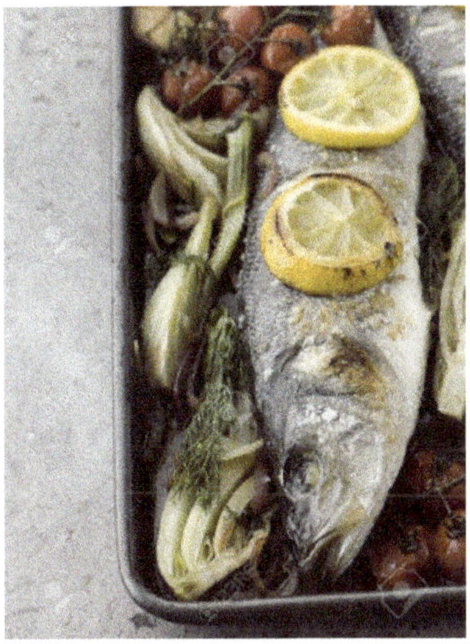

Preparation time:5 minutes

Cooking time:15 minutes

Servings:2

Ingredients:

- 1 lemon
- ½ sliced fennel bulb
- 6 oz. sea bass fillets
- 1 tsp. black pepper
- 2 garlic cloves

Directions:

1. Preheat the oven to 375°F/Gas Mark 5.
2. Sprinkle black pepper over the Sea Bass.
3. Slice the fennel bulb and garlic cloves.
4. Add 1 salmon fillet and half the fennel and garlic to one sheet of baking paper or tin foil.
5. Squeeze in 1/2 lemon juices.
6. Repeat for the other fillet.
7. Fold and add to the oven for 12-15 minutes or until fish is thoroughly cooked through.
8. Meanwhile, add boiling water to your couscous, cover and allow to steam.
9. Serve with your choice of rice or salad.

Nutrition:

Calories 221,

Protein 14 g,

Carbs 3 g,

Fat 2 g,

Sodium (Na) 119 mg,

Potassium (K) 398 mg,

Phosphorus 149 mg

54. Lemon, Garlic & Cilantro Tuna and Rice

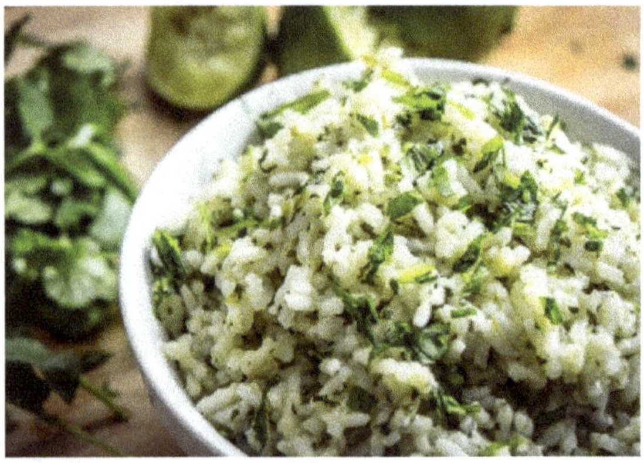

Preparation time:5 minutes

Cooking time:0 minutes

Servings:2

Ingredients:

- ½ cup arugula
- 1 tbsp. extra virgin olive oil
- 1 cup cooked rice
- 1 tsp. black pepper
- ¼ finely diced red onion
- 1 juiced lemon
- 3 oz. canned tuna
- 2 tbsps. Chopped fresh cilantro

Directions:

1. Mix the olive oil, pepper, cilantro and red onion in a bowl.
2. Stir in the tuna, cover and leave in the fridge for as long as possible (if you can) or serve immediately.
3. When ready to eat, serve up with the cooked rice and arugula!

Nutrition:

Calories 221,

Protein 11 g,

Carbs 26 g,

Fat 7 g,

Sodium (Na) 143 mg,

Potassium (K)197 mg,

Phosphorus 182 mg

55. Cod & Green Bean Risotto

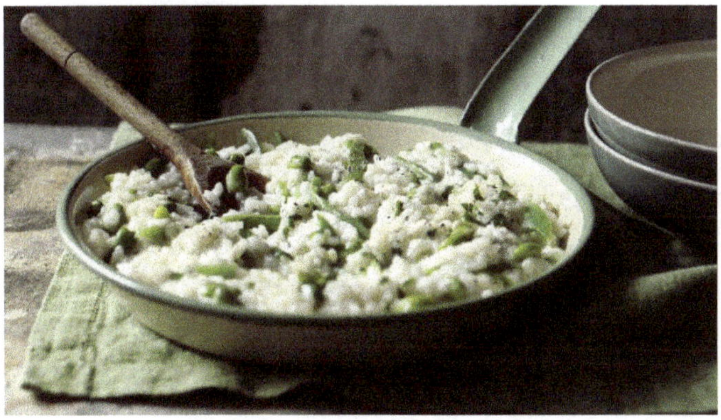

Preparation time:4 minutes

Cooking time:40 minutes

Servings:2

Ingredients:

- ½ cup arugula
- 1 finely diced white onion
- 4 oz. c od fillet
- 1 cup white rice

- 2 lemon wedges
- 1 cup boiling water
- ¼ tsp. black pepper
- 1 cup low sodium chicken broth
- 1 tbsp. extra virgin olive oil
- ½ cup green beans

Directions:

1. Heat the oil in a large pan on medium heat.
2. Sauté the chopped onion for 5 minutes until soft before adding in the rice and stirring for 1-2 minutes.
3. Combine the broth with boiling water.
4. Add half of the liquid to the pan and stir slowly.
5. Slowly add the rest of the liquid whilst continuously stirring for up to 20-30 minutes.
6. Stir in the green beans to the risotto.
7. Place the fish on top of the rice, cover and steam for 10 minutes.
8. Ensure the water does not dry out and keep topping up until the rice is cooked thoroughly.
9. Use your fork to break up the fish fillets and stir into the rice.
10. Sprinkle with freshly ground pepper to serve and a squeeze of fresh lemon.
11. Garnish with the lemon wedges and serve with the arugula.

Nutrition:

Calories 221,

Protein 12 g,

Carbs 29 g,

Fat 8 g,

Sodium (Na) 398 mg,

Potassium (K) 347 mg,

Phosphorus 241 mg

56. Sardine Fish Cakes

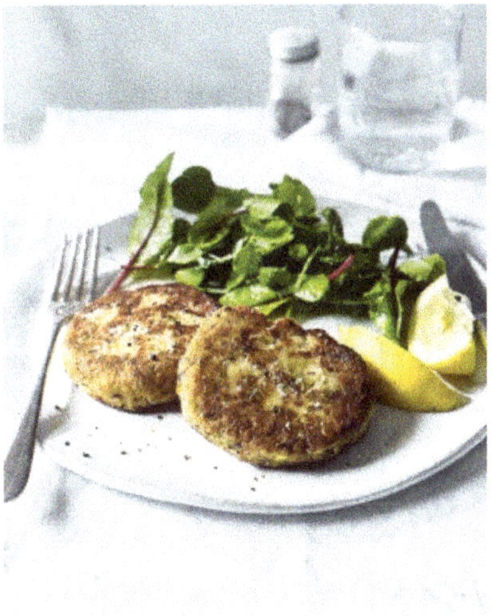

Preparation Time: 10 minutes

Cooking Time: 10 minutes

Servings:4

Ingredients:

- 11 oz sardines, canned, drained
- 1/3 cup shallot, chopped
- 1 teaspoon chili flakes
- ½ teaspoon salt
- 2 tablespoon wheat flour, whole grain
- 1 egg, beaten
- 1 tablespoon chives, chopped
- 1 teaspoon olive oil
- 1 teaspoon butter

Directions:

1. Put the butter in the skillet and melt it.
2. Add shallot and cook it until translucent.
3. After this, transfer the shallot in the mixing bowl.
4. Add sardines, chili flakes, salt, flour, egg, chives, and mix up until smooth with the help of the fork.
5. Make the medium size cakes and place them in the skillet.

6. Add olive oil.
7. Roast the fish cakes for 3 minutes from each side over the medium heat.
8. Dry the cooked fish cakes with the paper towel if needed and transfer in the serving plates.

Nutrition:

calories 221,

fat 12.2,

fiber 0.1,

carbs 5.4,

protein21.3

57. Cajun Catfish

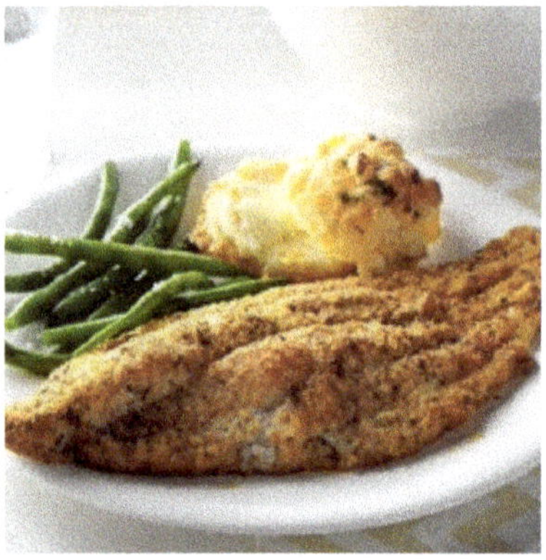

Preparation Time: 10 minutes

Cooking Time: 10 minutes

Servings:4

Ingredients:

- 16 oz catfish steaks (4 oz each fish steak)
- 1 tablespoon cajun spices
- 1 egg, beaten
- 1 tablespoon sunflower oil

Directions:

1. Pour sunflower oil in the skillet and preheat it until shimmering.
2. Meanwhile, dip every catfish steak in the beaten egg and coat in Cajun spices.

3. Place the fish steaks in the hot oil and roast them for 4 minutes from each side.
4. The cooked catfish steaks should have a light brown crust.

Nutrition:

calories 263,

fat 16.7,

fiber 0,

carbs 0.1,

protein 26.3

58. 4-Ingredients Salmon Fillet

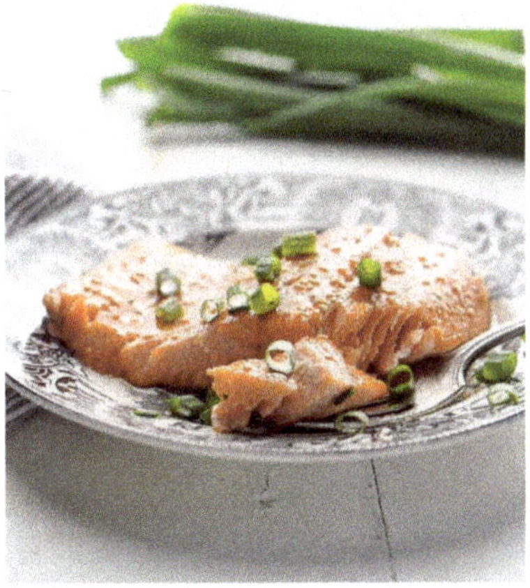

Preparation Time: 5 minutes

Cooking Time: 25 minutes

Servings:1

Ingredients:

- 4 oz salmon fillet
- ½ teaspoon salt
- 1 teaspoon sesame oil
- ½ teaspoon sage

Directions:

1. Rub the fillet with salt and sage.
2. Place the fish in the tray and sprinkle it with sesame oil.
3. Cook the fish for 25 minutes at 365F.
4. Flip the fish carefully onto another side after 12 minutes of cooking.

Nutrition:

calories 191,

fat 11.6,

fiber 0.1,

carbs 0.2,

protein 22

59. Spanish Cod in Sauce

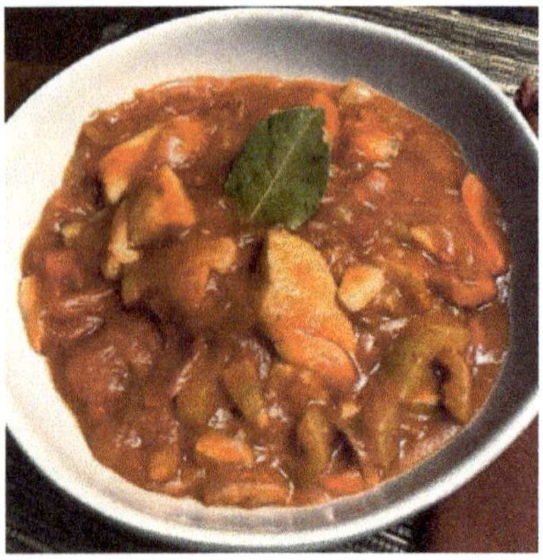

Preparation Time: 10 minutes

Cooking Time: 5.5 hours

Servings:2

Ingredients:

- 1 teaspoon tomato paste
- 1 teaspoon garlic, diced
- 1 white onion, sliced
- 1 jalapeno pepper, chopped
- 1/3 cup chicken stock
- 7 oz Spanish cod fillet

- 1 teaspoon paprika
- 1 teaspoon salt

Directions:

1. Pour chicken stock in the saucepan.
2. Add tomato paste and mix up the liquid until homogenous.
3. Add garlic, onion, jalapeno pepper, paprika, and salt.
4. Bring the liquid to boil and then simmer it.
5. Chop the cod fillet and add it in the tomato liquid.
6. Close the lid and simmer the fish for 10 minutes over the low heat.
7. Serve the fish in the bowls with tomato sauce.

Nutrition:

calories 113,

fat 1.2,

fiber 1.9,

carbs 7.2,

protein 18.9

60. Fish Shakshuka

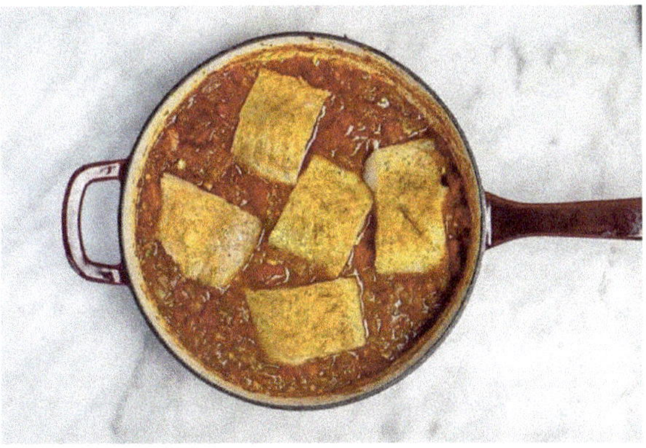

Preparation Time: 5 minutes

Cooking Time: 15 minutes

Servings:5

Ingredients:

- 5 eggs
- 1 cup tomatoes, chopped
- 3 bell peppers, chopped
- 1 tablespoon butter
- 1 teaspoon tomato paste
- 1 teaspoon chili pepper
- 1 teaspoon salt
- 1 tablespoon fresh dill
- 5 oz cod fillet, chopped
- 1 tablespoon scallions, chopped

Directions:

1. Melt butter in the skillet and add chili pepper, bell peppers, and tomatoes.
2. Sprinkle the vegetables with scallions, dill, salt, and chili pepper. Simmer them for 5 minutes.
3. After this, add chopped cod fillet and mix up well.
4. Close the lid and simmer the ingredients for 5 minutes over the medium heat.
5. Then crack the eggs over fish and close the lid.
6. Cook shakshuka with the closed lid for 5 minutes.

Nutrition:

calories 143,

fat 7.3,

fiber 1.6,

carbs 7.9,

protein12.8

61. Salmon Baked in Foil with Fresh Thyme

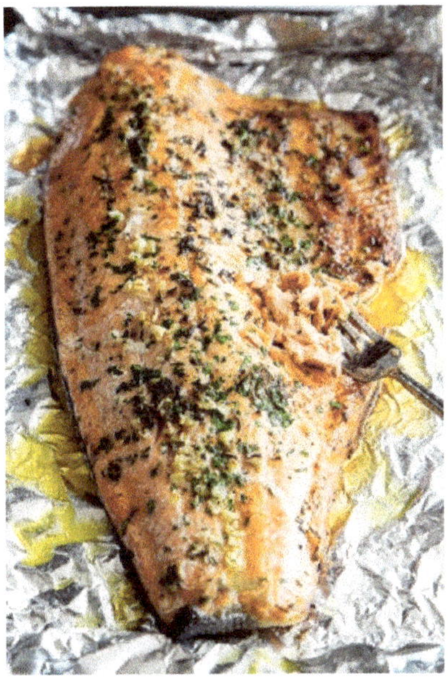

Preparation Time: 10 minutes

Cooking Time: 30 minutes

Servings:4

Ingredients:

- 4 fresh thyme sprig
- 4 garlic cloves, peeled, roughly chopped
- 16 oz salmon fillets (4 oz each fillet)
- ½ teaspoon salt
- ½ teaspoon ground black pepper
- 4 tablespoons cream
- 4 teaspoons butter
- ¼ teaspoon cumin seeds

Directions:

1. Line the baking tray with foil.
2. Sprinkle the fish fillets with salt, ground black pepper, cumin seeds, and arrange them in the tray with oil.
3. Add thyme sprig on the top of every fillet.
4. Then add cream, butter, and garlic.
5. Bake the fish for 30 minutes at 345F.

Nutrition:

calories 198,

fat 11.6,

fiber 0.2,

carbs 1.8,

protein 22.4

62. Poached Halibut in Orange Sauce

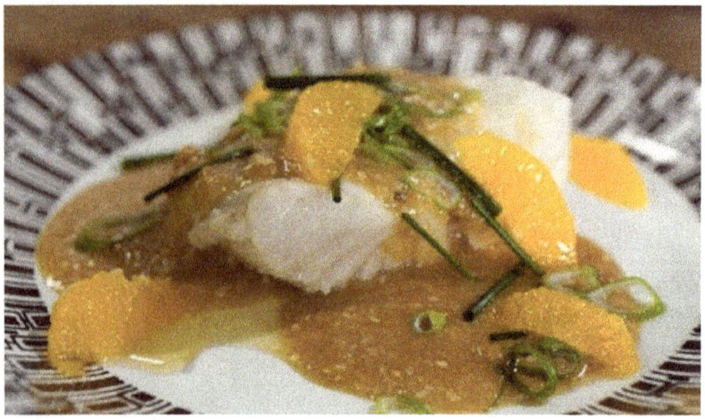

Preparation Time: 10 minutes

Cooking Time: 10 minutes

Servings: 4

Ingredients:

- 1-pound halibut
- 1/3 cup butter
- 1 rosemary sprig
- ½ teaspoon ground black pepper
- 1 teaspoon salt
- 1 teaspoon honey
- ¼ cup of orange juice
- 1 teaspoon cornstarch

Directions:

1. Put butter in the saucepan and melt it.
2. Add rosemary sprig.

3. Sprinkle the halibut with salt and ground black pepper.
4. Put the fish in the boiling butter and poach it for 4 minutes.
5. Meanwhile, pour orange juice in the skillet. Add honey and bring the liquid to boil.
6. Add cornstarch and whisk until the liquid will start to be thick.
7. Then remove it from the heat.
8. Transfer the poached halibut in the plate and cut it on 4.
9. Place every fish serving in the serving plate and top with orange sauce.

Nutrition:

calories 349,

fat 29.3,

fiber 0.1,

carbs 3.2,

protein 17.8

63. Fishen Papillote

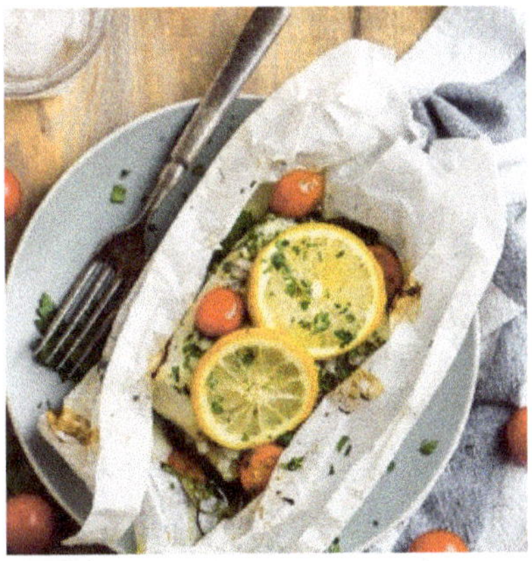

Preparation Time: 15 minutes

Cooking Time: 20 minutes

Servings:3

Ingredients:

- 10 oz snapper fillet
- 1 tablespoon fresh dill, chopped
- 1 white onion, peeled, sliced
- ½ teaspoon tarragon

- 1 tablespoon olive oil
- 1 teaspoon salt
- ½ teaspoon hot pepper
- 2 tablespoons sour cream

Directions:

1. Make the medium size packets from parchment and arrange them in the baking tray.
2. Cut the snapper fillet on 3 and sprinkle them with salt, tarragon, and hot pepper.
3. Put the fish fillets in the parchment packets.
4. Then top the fish with olive oil, sour cream sliced onion, and fresh dill.
5. Bake the fish for 20 minutes at 355F.

Nutrition:

calories 204,

fat 8.2,

fiber 1,

carbs 4.6,

protein 27.2

64. Tuna Casserole

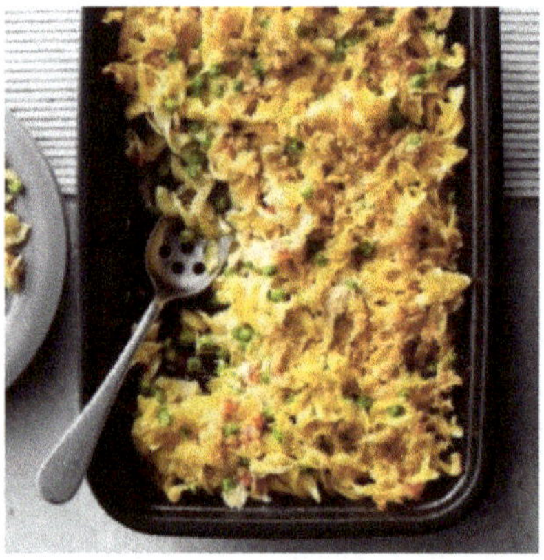

Preparation Time: 15 minutes

Cooking Time: 35 minutes

Servings:4

Ingredients:

- ½ cup Cheddar cheese, shredded
- 2 tomatoes, chopped
- 7 oz tuna filet, chopped
- 1 teaspoon ground coriander
- ½ teaspoon salt
- 1 teaspoon olive oil
- ½ teaspoon dried oregano

Directions:

1. Brush the casserole mold with olive oil.
2. Mix up together chopped tuna fillet with dried oregano and ground coriander.
3. Place the fish in the mold and flatten well to get the layer.
4. Then add chopped tomatoes and shredded cheese.
5. Cover the casserole with foil and secure the edges.
6. Bake the meal for 35 minutes at 355F.

Nutrition:

calories 260,

fat 21.5,

fiber 0.8,

carbs 2.7,

protein 14.6

65. Oregano Salmon with Crunchy Crust

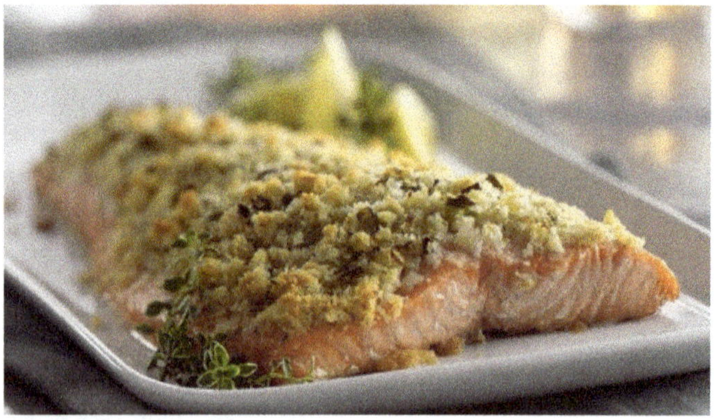

Preparation Time: 10 minutes

Cooking Time: 2 hours

Servings:2

Ingredients:

- 8 oz salmon fillet
- 2 tablespoons panko breadcrumbs
- 1 oz Parmesan, grated
- 1 teaspoon dried oregano
- 1 teaspoon sunflower oil

Directions:

1. In the mixing bowl combine together panko breadcrumbs, Parmesan, and dried oregano.
2. Sprinkle the salmon with olive oil and coat in the breadcrumb's mixture.
3. After this, line the baking tray with baking paper.
4. Place the salmon in the tray and transfer in the preheated to the 385F oven.
5. Bake the salmon for 25 minutes.

Nutrition:

calories 245,

fat 12.8,

fiber 0.6,

carbs 5.9,

protein 27.5

66. Baked Fish à la Mushrooms

Preparation Time: 10 minutes

Cooking Time: 17 minutes

Servings: 2

Ingredients:

- 1 lb. fresh cod fillets
- 2 tablespoons margarine
- 1-1/2 cups sliced fresh mushrooms
- 1/4 cup white onion
- 1 teaspoon dried thyme

Directions:

1. First place the fish fillets in a baking dish, suitable to fit the Instant Pot.
2. Melt margarine in a pan and add onion and mushroom.
3. Sauté this mixture for 5 minutes then pour over the fish.
4. Drizzle crushed thyme on top of the sauce.
5. Put 1.5 cups water into the Instant Pot and place a trivet over it.
6. Place the prepared baking dish over this trivet.
7. Put back the lid and cook for 12 minutes on Manual mode at High pressure.
8. Then release the pressure completely then remove the pot's lid.
9. Serve warm.

Nutrition:

Calories 155

Total Fats 7 g

Saturated Fat 1.4 g

Cholesterol 49 mg

Sodium 110 mg

Total Carbs 2 g

Fiber 0.5 g

Sugar 0.3 g

Protein 21 g

Chapter 14. Vegetarian Recipes

67. Egg White Frittata with Penne

Preparation Time: 15 minutes

Cooking Time: 30 minutes

Serving: 4

Ingredients:

- 6 egg whites
- ¼ cup rice milk
- 1 tablespoon chopped fresh parsley
- 1 teaspoon chopped fresh thyme
- 1 teaspoon chopped fresh chives
- Freshly ground black pepper
- 2 teaspoons olive oil
- ¼ small sweet onion, chopped
- 1 teaspoon minced garlic
- ½ cup boiled and chopped red bell pepper
- 2 cups cooked penne

Directions:

1. Heat the oven to 350°F.
2. In a container, whisk together the egg whites, rice milk, parsley, thyme, chives, and pepper.
3. Preheat the olive oil.
4. Sauté the onion, garlic, and red pepper for about 4 minutes or until they are softened.
5. Using a spatula, add the cooked penne to the skillet to evenly distribute the pasta.
6. Pour the egg mixture over the pasta and shake the pan to coat the pasta.
7. Leave the skillet on the heat for 1 minute to set the bottom of the frittata and then transfer the skillet to the oven.
8. Bake the frittata for about 25 minutes or until it is set and golden brown.
9. Remove from the oven and serve immediately.

Nutrition:

Calories: 170

Fat: 3g

Carbohydrates:25g

Phosphorus: 62mg

Potassium: 144mg

Sodium: 90mg

Protein: 10g

68. Vegetable Fried Rice

Preparation Time: 20 minutes

Cooking Time: 20 minutes

Serving: 6

Ingredients:

- 1 tablespoon olive oil
- ½ sweet onion, chopped
- 1 tablespoon grated fresh ginger
- 2 teaspoons minced garlic
- 1 cup sliced carrots
- ½ cup chopped eggplant
- ½ cup peas
- ½ cup green beans, cut into 1-inch pieces
- 2 tablespoons chopped fresh cilantro
- 3 cups cooked rice

Directions:

1. Over medium-high heat, heat the olive oil.
2. Sauté the onion, ginger, and garlic for about 3 minutes or until softened.
3. Stir in the carrot, eggplant, peas, and green beans and sauté for 3 minutes more.
4. Add the cilantro and rice.
5. Sauté, stirring constantly, for about 10 minutes or until the rice is heated through.

6. Serve immediately.

Nutrition:

Calories: 189

Fat: 7g

Carbohydrates: 28g

Phosphorus: 89mg

Potassium: 172mg

Sodium: 13mg

Protein: 6g

69. Bulgur-Stuffed Spaghetti Squash

Preparation Time: 20 minutes

Cooking Time: 50 minutes

Serving: 4

Ingredients:

FOR THE SQUASH

- 2 small spaghetti squash, halved
- 1 teaspoon olive oil
- Freshly ground black pepper

FOR THE FILLING

- 1 teaspoon olive oil
- ½ small sweet onion, finely diced
- 1 teaspoon minced garlic
- ½ cup chopped carrot
- ½ cup cranberries
- 1 teaspoon chopped fresh thyme
- ½ teaspoon ground cumin
- ½ teaspoon ground coriander
- Juice of ½ lemon
- 1 cup cooked bulgur

Directions:

TO MAKE THE SQUASH

1. Preheat the oven to 350°F.
2. Line a baking sheet with parchment paper.
3. Grease the cut sides of the squash, season with pepper, and place them cut-side down on the baking sheet.
4. Bake for 25 to 30 min until it become tender. Remove the squash from the oven and flip the squash halves over.
5. Scoop the flesh from each half, leaving about ½ inch around the edges and keeping the skin intact.
6. Place 2 cups of squash flesh in a large bowl and reserve the rest for another recipe.

TO MAKE THE FILLING

1. Heat the olive oil.
2. Sauté the onion, garlic, carrot, and cranberries for 5 to 6 minutes or until softened.
3. Add the sautéed vegetables to the squash in the bowl.
4. Add the thyme, cumin, and coriander, stirring to combine.
5. Stir in the lemon juice and cooked bulgur until well mixed.
6. Spoon the filling evenly into the squash halves.
7. Bake for about 15 min or until heated through.
8. Serve warm.

Nutrition:

Calories: 111

Fat: 2g

Carbohydrates: 17g

Phosphorus: 38mg

Potassium: 182mg

Sodium: 22mg

Protein: 3g

70. Red Pepper Strata

Preparation Time: 20 minutes,

Cooking Time: 1 hour, 5 minutes

Serving: 8

Ingredients:

- Butter, for greasing the baking dish
- 8 slices fresh white bread, cut into cubes
- 1 tablespoon unsalted butter
- ½ sweet onion, chopped
- 1 teaspoon minced garlic
- 1 red bell pepper, boiled and chopped
- 6 eggs
- ¼ cup tarragon vinegar
- 1 cup rice milk
- 1 teaspoon Tabasco sauce
- ½ teaspoon freshly ground black pepper
- 1 ounce Parmesan cheese, grated

Directions:

1. Preheat the oven to 250°F.
2. Grease a 9-by-9-inch baking dish with butter; set aside.
3. Layer the baking sheet with parchment paper and scatter the bread cubes on the sheet.
4. Bake the bread cubes until they are crisp.
5. Remove the bread cubes from the oven then set aside.
6. Over medium-high heat, melt the butter.
7. Sauté the onion and garlic for about 3 minutes or until softened.
8. Add the red pepper and sauté an additional 2 minutes.
9. Spread half of the bread cubes in a layer in the baking dish and top with half of the sautéed vegetables.
10. Repeat with the remaining half of the bread cubes and vegetables.
11. In a medium bowl, whisk together the eggs, vinegar, rice milk, hot sauce, and pepper.
12. Put the egg mixture evenly into the baking dish.
13. Cover the dish and place in the fridge to soak for at least 2 hours or overnight.
14. Let the strata come to room temperature.
15. Preheat the oven to 325°F.
16. Remove the plastic wrap and bake for about 45 minutes or until golden.
17. Sprinkle the top of the strata with cheese and bake an additional 5 minutes.

18. Serve hot.

Nutrition:

Calories: 150

Fat: 6g

Carbohydrates: 10g

Phosphorus: 120mg

Potassium: 89mg

Sodium: 168mg

Protein: 7g

71. Couscous Burgers

Preparation Time: 20 minutes, plus 1-hour chilling time

Cooking Time: 10 minutes

Serving: 4

Ingredients:

- ½ cup canned chickpeas, rinsed and drained
- 2 tablespoons chopped fresh cilantro
- 2 tablespoons chopped fresh parsley
- 1 tablespoon freshly squeezed lemon juice
- 2 teaspoons lemon zest
- 1 teaspoon minced garlic
- 2½ cups cooked couscous
- 2 eggs, lightly beaten
- 2 tablespoons olive oil

Directions:

1. Combine the chickpeas, cilantro, parsley, lemon juice, lemon zest, and garlic in a food processor and pulse until a paste forms (or use a large bowl and a handheld immersion blender).
2. Put the the chickpea mixture to a bowl and add the couscous and eggs, mixing thoroughly to combine.

3. Chill the mixture in the refrigerator for 1 hour to firm it.
4. Form the couscous mixture into 4 patties.
5. Place a large skillet over medium-high heat and add the olive oil.
6. Place the patties in the skillet, 2 at a time, gently pressing them down with the back of a spatula. Cook for 5 minutes or until golden, and flip the patties over.
7. Cook the other side for 5 minutes and transfer the cooked burgers to a plate covered with a paper towel.
8. Repeat with the remaining 2 burgers.

Nutrition:

Calories: 242

Fat: 10g

Carbohydrates: 29g

Phosphorus: 108mg

Potassium: 168mg

Sodium: 43mg

Protein: 9g

72. Marinated Tofu Stir-Fry

Preparation Time: 20 minutes

Cooking Time: 20 minutes

Serving: 4

Ingredients:

For the tofu

- 1 tablespoon freshly squeezed lemon juice
- 1 teaspoon minced garlic
- 1 teaspoon grated fresh ginger
- Pinch red pepper flakes
- 5 ounces extra-firm tofu, pressed well and cubed (see ingredient tip)

For the stir-fry

- 1 tablespoon olive oil

- ½ cup cauliflower florets
- ½ cup thinly sliced carrots
- ½ cup julienned red pepper
- ½ cup fresh green beans
- 2 cups cooked white rice

Directions:

To make the tofu

1. Combine together the lemon juice, garlic, ginger, and red pepper flakes.
2. Add the tofu and toss it around for coating.
3. Place the bowl in the refrigerator and marinate for 2 hours.

To make the stir fry

1. Heat the oil.
2. Sauté the tofu for about 8 minutes or until it is lightly browned and heated through.
3. Add the cauliflower and carrots and sauté for 5 minutes, stirring and tossing constantly.
4. Add the red pepper and green beans; sauté for 3 additional minutes.
5. Serve over the white rice.

Ingredient tip: Draining tofu is a crucial step to ensure this porous product absorbs all the flavor in the dish. Drench the oil of the tofu on a paper towel-lined plate and cover the block with more paper towels. Set something heavy such as a large can or a book on the tofu. Check the drainage every 30 minutes, changing the paper towels if needed, for two hours.

Dialysis modification: Omit the red peppers from the dish to lower the amount of potassium in the recipe.

Nutrition:

Calories: 190

Fat: 6g

Carbohydrates: 30g

Phosphorus: 90mg

Potassium: 199mg

Sodium: 22mg

Protein: 6g

73. Thai-Inspired Vegetable Curry

Preparation Time: 15 minutes

Cooking Time: 45 minutes

Serving: 4

Ingredients:

- 2 teaspoons olive oil
- ½ sweet onion, diced
- 2 teaspoons minced garlic
- 2 teaspoons grated fresh ginger
- ½ eggplant, peeled and diced
- 1 carrot, peeled and diced
- 1 red bell pepper, diced
- 1 tablespoon Hot Curry Powder
- 1 teaspoon ground cumin
- ½ teaspoon coriander
- Pinch cayenne pepper
- 1½ cups homemade vegetable stock
- 1 tablespoon cornstarch
- ¼ cup water

Directions:

1. Over medium-high heat, heat the oil.
2. Sauté the onion, garlic, and ginger for 3 minutes or until they are softened.
3. Add the eggplant, carrots, and red pepper, and sauté, stirring often, for 6 additional minutes.
4. Stir in the curry powder, cumin, coriander, cayenne pepper, and vegetable stock.
5. Put the curry to a boil and then reduce the heat to low.
6. Simmer the curry for about 30 minutes or until the vegetables are tender.
7. Stir together the cornstarch and water.
8. Mix the cornstarch mixture into the curry and simmer for about 5 minutes or until the sauce is thickened.

Nutrition:

Calories: 100

Fat: 3g

Carbohydrates: 9g

Phosphorus: 28mg

Potassium: 180mg

Sodium: 218mg

Protein: 1g

74. Linguine With Roasted Red Pepper–Basil Sauce

Preparation Time: 20 minutes

Cooking Time: 20 minutes

Serving: 4

Ingredients:

- 8 ounces uncooked linguine
- 1 teaspoon olive oil
- ½ sweet onion, chopped
- 2 teaspoons minced garlic
- 1 cup chopped roasted red bell peppers
- 1 teaspoon balsamic vinegar
- ¼ cup shredded fresh basil
- Pinch red pepper flakes
- Freshly ground black pepper
- 4 teaspoons grated low-fat Parmesan cheese, for garnish

Directions:

1. Cook the pasta y following the package instructions.
2. While the pasta is cooking, place a large skillet over medium-high heat and add the olive oil.
3. Sauté the onions and garlic for about 3 minutes or until they are softened.
4. Add the red pepper, vinegar, basil, and red pepper flakes to the skillet and stir for about 5 minutes or until heated through.

5. Mix the cooked pasta with the sauce and season with pepper.
6. Serve topped with Parmesan cheese.

Nutrition:

Calories: 246

Fat: 3g

Carbohydrates: 41g

Phosphorus: 117mg

Potassium: 187mg

Sodium: 450mg

Protein: 13g

75. Baked Mac and Cheese

Preparation Time: 10 minutes

Cooking Time: 25 minutes

Serving: 4

Ingredients:

- 1 teaspoon olive oil
- ½ sweet onion, chopped
- 1 teaspoon minced garlic
- ¼ cup rice milk
- 1 cup cream cheese
- ½ teaspoon dry mustard
- ½ teaspoon freshly ground black pepper
- Pinch cayenne pepper
- 3 cups cooked macaroni

Directions:

1. Preheat the oven to 375°F.
2. Grease a 9-by-9-inch baking dish with butter; set aside.
3. In a medium saucepan over medium heat, heat the olive oil.

4. Sauté the onion and garlic for about 3 minutes or until softened.
5. Stir in the milk, cheese, mustard, black pepper, and cayenne pepper until the mixture is smooth and well blended.
6. Add the cooked macaroni, stirring to coat.
7. Transfer the mixture into a baking dish and place in the oven.
8. Bake for about 15 minutes or until the macaroni is bubbly.

Dialysis modification: This dish is rich, so you can choose a smaller portion size to reduce your phosphorus and potassium intake.

Nutrition:

Calories: 386

Fat: 22g

Carbohydrates: 37g

Phosphorus: 120mg

Potassium: 146mg

Sodium: 219mg

Protein: 10g

76. Grilled Kale and Fried Egg On Bread

Preparation Time: 10 minutes

Cooking Time: 20 minutes

Serving: 2

Ingredients:

- 2 medium kale leaves
- ½ teaspoon olive oil
- Pinch red pepper flakes
- 4 teaspoons unsalted butter, divided
- 2 slices white bread
- 2 teaspoons cream cheese
- 2 small eggs
- Freshly ground black pepper

Directions:

1. Preheat the oven to 350°F.
2. Mix the kale leaves with the olive oil until they are completely coated.
3. Sprinkle a pinch of red pepper flakes over the kale leaves.
4. Place the leaves in a pie plate and roast for about 10 minutes or until crispy.
5. Remove the kale from the oven; set aside.
6. Butter both sides of the bread with 1 teaspoon butter per slice.
7. Toast the bread on both sides for about 3 minutes or until it is golden brown.
8. Transfer the bread from the skillet and spread 1 teaspoon cream cheese on each slice.
9. Melt the remaining 2 teaspoons of butter in the skillet and fry the eggs sunny-side up, for about 4 minutes.
10. Place a piece of crispy kale and a fried egg on top of each slice of the cream cheese–topped bread.
11. Serve seasoned with pepper.

Nutrition:

Calories: 224

Fat: 15g

Carbohydrates: 14g

Phosphorus: 118mg

Potassium: 175mg

Sodium: 200mg

Protein: 8g

77. Tofu and Eggplant Stir-Fry

Preparation Time: 20 minutes

Cooking Time: 20 minutes

Serving: 4

Ingredients:

- 1 tablespoon granulated sugar
- 1 tablespoon all-purpose flour
- 1 teaspoon grated fresh ginger
- 1 teaspoon minced garlic

- 1 teaspoon minced jalapeño pepper
- Juice of 1 lime
- Water
- 2 tablespoons olive oil, divided
- 5 ounces extra-firm tofu, cut into ½-inch cubes
- 2 cups cubed eggplant
- 2 scallions
- 3 tablespoons chopped cilantro

Directions:

1. Combine together the sugar, flour, ginger, garlic, jalapeño, lime juice, and enough water to make 2/3 cup of sauce then set aside.
2. In a large skillet over medium-high heat, heat 1 tablespoon of the oil.
3. Sauté the tofu for about 6 minutes or until it is crisp and golden.
4. Remove the tofu; set aside on a plate.
5. Add the remaining 1 tablespoon oil and sauté the eggplant cubes for about 10 minutes or until they look golde brown.
6. Add the tofu and scallions to the skillet and toss to combine.
7. Mix in the sauce and bring to a boil, stirring constantly, for about 2 minutes or until the sauce is thickened.
8. Add the cilantro before serving.

Nutrition:

Calories: 386

Fat: 22g

Carbohydrates: 37g

Phosphorus: 120mg

Potassium: 146mg

Sodium: 219mg

Protein: 10g

78. Mie Goreng with Broccoli

Preparation Time: 10 minutes, plus 30 minutes draining time

Cooking Time: 20 minutes

Serving: 4

Ingredients:

- ½ pound rice noodles
- ¼ cup packed dark brown sugar
- 2 teaspoons minced garlic
- 1 teaspoon grated fresh ginger
- 1 teaspoon low-sodium soy sauce
- ½ teaspoon sambal oelek
- 4 ounces extra-firm tofu, cut into ½-inch cubes
- 1 tablespoon cornstarch
- 2 tablespoons olive oil, divided
- 2 cups broccoli, cut into small size
- 2 scallions, both green and white parts, sliced thin on the diagonal
- Lime wedges, for garnish

Directions:

1. Cook the noodles by following the package instructions; drain and set aside.
2. In a small bowl, whisk together the brown sugar, garlic, ginger, soy sauce, and sambal oelek; set aside.
3. Drain the tofu on paper towels for 30 minutes and pat the tofu dry.
4. Toss the tofu with the cornstarch and shake to remove the excess.
5. Heat 1 tablespoon of the olive oil over medium heat.
6. Add the tofu and sauté for about 10 minutes or until the tofu is browned on all sides and crispy.
7. Put the tofu to a plate with a slotted spoon.
8. Add the 1 tablespoon oil to the skillet.
9. Sauté the broccoli for about 4 minutes or until it is tender.
10. Add the sauce and tofu to the skillet and cook for about 2 minutes or until the sauce thickens.
11. Serve topped with scallions and garnish with lime wedges.

Nutrition:

Calories: 360

Fat: 11g

Carbohydrates: 62g

Phosphorus: 120mg

Potassium: 193mg

Sodium: 166mg

Protein: 4g

79. Spicy Veggie Pancakes

Preparation Time: 20 minutes

Cooking Time: 10 minutes

Serving: 4

Ingredients:

- 3 tablespoons olive oil, divided
- 2 small onions, finely chopped
- 1 jalapeño pepper, minced
- ¾ cup carrot, grated
- ¾ cup cabbage, finely chopped
- 1½ cups quick-cooking oats
- ¾ cup cooked brown rice
- ¾ cup water
- ½ cup whole-wheat flour
- 1 large egg
- 1 large egg white
- 1 teaspoon baking soda
- ¼ teaspoon cayenne pepper

Directions:

1. Heat 2 teaspoons oil over medium heat.
2. Sauté the onion, jalapeño, carrot, and cabbage for 4 minutes.

3. While the veggies are cooking, combine the oats, rice, water, flour, egg, egg white, baking soda, and pepper in a mixing bowl.

4. Add the cooked vegetables to the mixture and stir to combine.

5. Heat the remaining oil in a pan over medium heat.

6. Drop the mixture into the skillet, about 1/3 cup per pancake. Cook for 4 minutes until bubbles form on the surface of the pancakes and the edges look cooked, then carefully flip them over.

7. Cook the second sides for 3 to 5 minutes or until the pancakes are hot and firm.

8. Repeat with the remaining mixture and serve.

Make It Easier Tip: To save on prep time, purchase pre-grated carrots and cabbage. Brown rice can also be bought frozen and then microwaved according to package directions when you're ready to use it.

Nutrition:

Calories: 323

Total fat 11g

Saturated fat 2g

Sodium: 366mg

Potassium: 381mg

Phosphorus: 263mg

Carbohydrates: 48g

Fiber: 7g

Protein: 10g

80. Egg and Veggie Fajitas

Preparation Time: 20 minutes

Cooking Time: 10 minutes

Serving: 4

Ingredients:

- 3 large eggs
- 3 egg whites
- 2 teaspoons chili powder
- 1 tablespoon unsalted butter

- 1 onion, chopped
- 2 garlic cloves, minced
- 1 jalapeño pepper, minced
- 1 red bell pepper, chopped
- 1 cup frozen corn, thawed and drained
- 8 (6-inch) corn tortillas

Directions:

1. Whisk the eggs, egg whites, and chili powder in a small bowl until well combined. Set aside.
2. Melt the butter over medium heat.
3. Sauté the onion, garlic, jalapeño, bell pepper, and corn, until the vegetables are tender, 3 to 4 minutes.
4. Put in the the beaten egg mixture to the skillet. Cook, stirring occasionally, until the eggs form large curds and are set, 3 to 5 minutes.
5. Meanwhile, soften the corn tortillas as directed on the package.
6. Divide the egg mixture evenly among the softened corn tortillas. Roll the tortillas up and serve.

Increase Protein Tip: To make this a medium-protein recipe, increase the egg whites to 6 and replace 1 cup frozen corn with 1 cup canned no-salt-added or low-sodium canned black beans. The protein will increase to 19 grams.

Nutrition:

Calories: 316

Total fat 14g

Saturated fat: 3g

Sodium: 167mg

Potassium: 408mg

Phosphorus: 287mg

Carbohydrates: 35g

Fiber: 5g

Protein: 14g

Sugar: 4g

81. Pesto Pasta Salad

Preparation Time: 15 minutes

Cooking Time: 15 minutes

Servings: 5

Ingredients:

- 1 cup fresh basil leaves
- ½ cup packed fresh flat-leaf parsley leaves
- ½ cup arugula, chopped
- 2 tablespoons Parmesan cheese, grated
- ¼ cup extra-virgin olive oil
- 3 tablespoons mayonnaise
- 2 tablespoons water
- 12 ounces whole-wheat rotini pasta
- 1 red bell pepper, chopped
- 1 medium yellow summer squash, sliced
- 1 cup frozen baby peas

Directions:

1. Bring a large pot of water to boil.
2. Meanwhile, combine the basil, parsley, arugula, cheese, and olive oil in a blender or food processor. Blend until the herbs are finely chopped. Add the mayonnaise and water, then process again. Set aside.
3. Put the pasta to the pot of boiling water; cook according to package directions, about 8 to 9 minutes. Drain well, reserving ¼ cup of the cooking liquid.
4. Combine the pesto, pasta, bell pepper, squash, and peas in a large bowl and toss gently, adding enough of the reserved pasta cooking liquid to make a sauce on the salad. Serve immediately or cover and chill, then serve.
5. Store in an airtight container and refrigerate up to 3 days.

Ingredient Tip: Since you don't cook the extra-virgin olive oil in this recipe, a good quality brand will contribute increased flavor and richness. Reserve the more expensive, higher quality extra-virgin olive oil for recipes like this one and stick to using regular olive oil for sautéing.

Nutrition:

Calories: 378

Total fat 24g

Saturated fat: 4g

Sodium: 163mg

Potassium: 472mg

Phosphorus: 213mg

Carbohydrates: 35

Fiber: 6g

Protein: 9g

Sugar: 5g

82. Eggplant Casserole

Preparation Time: 10 minutes

Cooking Time: 20 minutes

Servings: 4

Ingredients:

- 3 cups eggplant
- 3 large eggs
- 1/2 cup liquid nondairy creamer
- 1/2 teaspoons black pepper
- 1/4 teaspoons sage
- 1/2 cup breadcrumbs
- 1 tablespoon margarine

Directions:

1. First, boil the eggplant in a saucepan filled with water until soft.
2. Drain and mash the eggplant in a bowl.
3. Now beat the eggs with black pepper, cream, sage, and eggplant mash.
4. Spread this mixture over the surface of the a baking dish and top it with breadcrumbs and butter.
5. Pour 1.5 cups of water into the Instant pot and set the trivet over it.

6. Place the baking dish over the trivet.
7. Seal the lid and cook for 15 minutes on Manual mode at High pressure.
8. Then, release the pressure completely then remove the pot's lid.
9. Broil this casserole for 5 minutes in the oven at Broiler settings.
    i. Serve warm.

Nutrition:

Calories 186

Total Fats 9 g

Saturated Fat 0.4 g

Cholesterol 124 mg

Sodium 246 mg

Total Carbs 19 g

Fiber 1.9 g

Sugar 1.2 g

Protein 7 g

Chapter 15. Vegan Recipes

83. Sweet Potato Chili

Preparation time: 5 minutes

Cooking Time: 4 hours

Servings: 1

Ingredients:

- 1 onion
- 1 bunch fresh coriander
- 1 yellow pepper
- 2 red peppers
- 1 fresh red chili
- 2 sweet potatoes, skin removed, chopped
- 2 tsp. ground cinnamon
- 1 tbsp. ground cumin
- 1 tsp. smoked paprika
- ½ cup water

Directions:

1. Layer chopped sweet potato inside the slow cooker. Sprinkle cumin, paprika, and cinnamon.
2. Add in onion, coriander, yellow peppers, red peppers, and red chili. Pour ½ cup of water.
3. Seal the lid and cook for 4 hours on low. Secure the lid.
4. After the 4-hour cooking cycle, turn off the heat. Adjust seasoning according to your preferred taste.
5. Serve over rice and guacamole on the side.

Nutrition:

Protein: 12.0 g

Potassium: 180 mg

Sodium: 120 mg

84. Hulled Barley with Veggies

Preparation time: 5 minutes

Cooking Time: 4 hours

Servings: 1

Ingredients:

- ¼ cup carrot, diced
- ¼ cup corn kernels
- ¼ cup green onion, sliced thinly
- ¾ cup barley, hulled
- ½ tsp. garlic powder
- 2 cups vegetable broth
- ¼ cup green beans, chopped
- ½ tsp. dried thyme
- ½ tbsp. nutritional yeast
- ¾ tsp. dill weed
- ¼ tsp. ground black pepper

Directions:

1. Place barley inside the slow cooker. Pour vegetable broth and pepper to the barley. Stir mixture well.
2. Add in carrot, corn, nutritional yeast, weed, dill, thyme, and garlic powder. Mix well.
3. Cover and cook for 2 hours on low. Secure the lid.
4. After the 2-hour cooking cycle, turn off the heat. Adjust seasoning according to your preferred taste. Serve.

Nutrition:

Protein: 23.0 g

Potassium: 25.7 mg

Sodium: 22.1 mg

85. Salmon Chowder

Preparation time: 5 minutes

Cooking Time: 4 hours

Servings: 2

Ingredients:

- 3 lbs salmon fillets, sliced into manageable pieces
- 1 1/2 cups onion, chopped
- 2 potatoes, cubed – limit this
- 3 cups water
- 1/3 tsp pepper
- 18 oz evaporated milk, non-fat

Directions:

1. Put together onion, salmon, potatoes, and pepper in the slow cooker. Pour water
2. Seal the lid and cook for 8 hours on low.
3. After the 8-hour cooking cycle, turn off the heat. Adjust seasoning according to your preferred taste.
4. Stir in milk. Cover and cook for another 30 minutes. Serve right away.

Nutrition:

Protein: 33.8 g

Potassium: 204.3 mg

Sodium: 183.5 mg

86. Beef Stew Pasta

Preparation time: 5 minutes

Cooking Time: 8 hours

Servings: 2

Ingredients:

- 1 Tbsp. olive oil

- 3/4 lb beef round roast, sliced into bite-sized pieces
- 1/2 cup onion, chopped
- 1/2 cup carrots, chopped
- 1/2 cup celery, chopped
- 2 cups beef broth, no salt
- 1/2 tsp oregano
- 1/4 cup red wine
- 1/4 tsp thyme
- 1/4 tsp black pepper
- 2 small tomatoes, diced – limit this
- 1/4 cup whole wheat pasta

Directions:

1. Pour olive oil into non-stick skillet. Cook beef round roast, in batches, for 5 minutes or until browned all over. Transfer meat to the slow cooker.
2. Add in onion, tomatoes, carrots, celery, beef broth, oregano, red wine, thyme, black pepper, and pasta. Stir mixture well.
3. Seal the lid and cook for 8 hours on low.
4. After the 8-hour cooking cycle, turn off the heat. Adjust seasoning according to your preferred taste.
5. To serve, place pasta into plates. Pour sauce all over.

Nutrition:

Protein: 12.8 g

Potassium: 128.5mg

Sodium: 95.8 mg

87. Curried Veggies and Rice

Preparation Time: 13 minutes

Cooking Time: 18 minutes

Serving: 4

Ingredients:

- ¼ cup olive oil
- 1 cup long-grain white basmati rice
- 4 garlic cloves, minced
- 2½ teaspoons curry powder
- ½ cup sliced shiitake mushrooms
- 1 red bell pepper, chopped
- 1 cup frozen, shelled edamame
- 2 cups low-sodium vegetable broth
- 1/8 teaspoon freshly ground black pepper

Directions:

1. Preheat the olive oil in a large saucepan over medium heat.
2. Add the rice, garlic, curry powder, mushrooms, bell pepper, and edamame; cook, stirring, for 2 minutes.
3. Add the broth and black pepper and bring to a boil.
4. Reduce the heat to low, partially cover the pot, and simmer for 15 to 18 minutes or until the rice is tender. Stir and serve.

Increase Protein Tip: To make this a medium-protein recipe, beat 4 eggs, and add them to the rice mixture. Let it sit for 3 to 4 minutes until the eggs are cooked and set, then stir to mix the eggs through the rice. The protein content will increase to 15 grams.

Nutrition:

Calories: 347

Total fat: 16g

Saturated fat: 2g

Sodium: 114mg

Phosphorus: 131mg

Potassium: 334mg

Carbohydrates: 44g

Fiber: 4g

Protein: 8g

Sugar: 3g

88. Spicy Mushroom Stir- Fry

Preparation Time: 15 minutes

Cooking Time: 10 minutes

Servings: 5

Ingredients:

- 1 cup low-sodium vegetable broth
- 2 tablespoons cornstarch
- 1 teaspoon low-sodium soy sauce
- ½ teaspoon ground ginger
- 1/8 teaspoon cayenne pepper
- 2 tablespoons olive oil
- 2 (8-ounce) packages sliced button mushrooms
- 1 red bell pepper, chopped
- 1 jalapeño pepper, minced
- 3 cups brown rice that has been cooked in unsalted water
- 2 tablespoons sesame oil

Directions:

1. Whisk together the broth, cornstarch, soy sauce, ginger, and cayenne pepper and set aside.
2. Preheat the olive oil in a wok or heavy skillet over high heat.
3. Add the mushrooms and peppers and stir-fry for 3 to 5 minutes or until the vegetables are tender-crisp.
4. Stir the broth mixture patiently and add it to the wok; stir-fry for 3 to 5 minutes longer and the sauce has thickened. Serve the stir-fry over the hot cooked brown rice and drizzle with the sesame oil.

Ingredient Tip: If you don't like spicy food, feel free to omit or reduce the amount of jalapeño pepper and cayenne pepper used in this recipe.

Nutrition:

Calories: 361

Total fat: 16g

Saturated fat: 2g

Sodium: 95mg

Phosphorus: 267mg

Potassium: 582mg

Carbohydrates: 49g

Fiber: 4g

Protein: 8g

Sugar: 4g

89. Vegetable Biryani

Preparation Time: 20 minutes

Cooking Time: 10 minutes

Serving: 4

Ingredients:

- 2 tablespoons olive oil
- 1 onion, diced
- 4 garlic cloves, minced
- 1 tablespoon grated fresh ginger root
- 1 cup carrot, grated
- 2 cups chopped cauliflower
- 1 cup frozen baby peas
- 2 teaspoons curry powder
- 1 cup low-sodium vegetable broth
- 3 cups frozen cooked brown rice

Directions:

1. Preheat the olive oil over medium heat.
2. Add the onion, garlic, and ginger root and sauté, stirring frequently, until tender-crisp, 2 minutes.

3. Add the carrot, cauliflower, peas, and curry powder and cook for 2 minutes longer.

4. Stir in the vegetable broth evenly and bring to a simmer. Reduce the heat to low, partially cover the skillet, and simmer for 6 to 7 minutes or until the vegetables are tender.

5. Meanwhile, heat the rice as directed on the package.

6. Stir the rice into the vegetable mixture and serve.

Nutrition:

Calories: 378

Total fat 16g

Saturated fat: 2g

Sodium: 113mg

Potassium: 510mg

Phosphorus: 236mg

Carbohydrates: 53g

Fiber: 7g

Protein: 8g

Sugar: 6g

90. Tex-Mex Pepper Stir- Fry

Preparation Time: 20 minutes

Cooking Time: 10 minutes

Serving: 3

Ingredients:

- 1/8 teaspoon cayenne pepper with the beans.
- 2 tablespoons olive oil
- 1 onion, chopped
- 4 garlic cloves, minced
- 1 jalapeño pepper, minced
- 1 red bell pepper, chopped
- 1 yellow bell pepper, chopped
- 1 cup canned no-salt-added or low-sodium black beans, rinsed and drained

- ½ cup powerhouse salsa
- Juice from 1 lemon
- 2 cups cooked brown rice

Directions:

1. Preheat the oil in a large wok or skillet over medium-high heat.
2. Add the onion and garlic and stir-fry for 2 minutes.
3. Stir in the jalapeño pepper, red bell pepper, and yellow bell pepper, and stir-fry for another 3 minutes.
4. Add the black beans and stir-fry for 3 to 5 minutes longer or until the ingredients are heated through.
5. Stir in the salsa and lemon juice and serve over the rice.

Make It Easier Tip: Frozen mixed red bell peppers are available in most supermarkets, so you can use 2 cups of this product instead of fresh pepper to save prep time.

Nutrition:

Calories: 297

Total fat 8g

Saturated fat: 1g

Sodium: 29mg

Potassium: 589mg

Phosphorus: 212mg

Carbohydrates: 49g

Fiber: 9g

Protein: 8g

Sugar: 7g

91. Veggie Cabbage Stir- Fry

Preparation Time: 20 minutes

Cooking Time: 10 minutes

Serving: 4

Ingredients:

- 1 cup low-sodium vegetable broth
- 1 tablespoon cornstarch
- 2 teaspoons low-sodium soy sauce
- ½ teaspoon ground ginger
- 2 tablespoons olive oil
- 4 cups chopped cabbage
- 1 (8-ounce) package sliced mushrooms
- 2 cups grated carrots
- 2 garlic cloves, sliced
- 3 cups cooked brown rice

Directions:

1. Stir together the broth, cornstarch, soy sauce, and ginger; set aside.
2. Preheat the olive oil in a large skillet over medium heat.
3. Stir-fry the cabbage for 3 minutes.
4. Stir in the mushrooms, carrots, and garlic and stir-fry for another 2 minutes.
5. Add the broth mixture to the skillet. Stir until the sauce bubbles and thickens and the cabbage is tender, 4 to 5 minutes.
6. Serve the stir-fry over the rice.

Make It Easier Tip: To save time, you can use pre-shredded cabbage from the produce aisle in the supermarket. This product cooks more quickly, so only stir-fry for 1 minute in step 3.

Nutrition:

Calories: 307

Total fat 9g

Saturated fat: 1g

Sodium: 174mg

Potassium: 579mg

Phosphorus: 247mg

Carbohydrates: 52g

Fiber: 6g

Protein: 8g

Sugar: 6g

92. Italian Chicken Stew

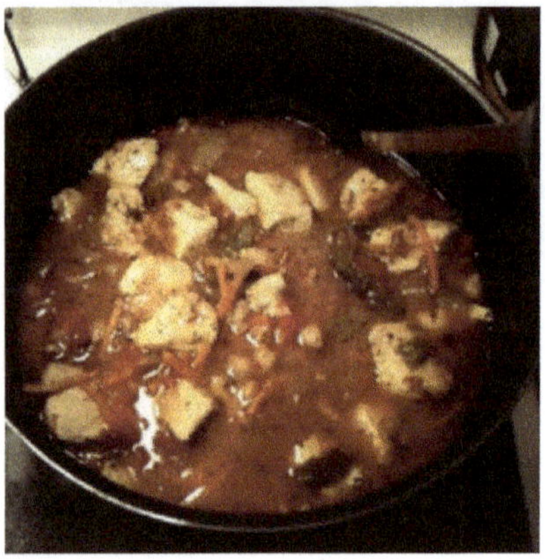

Preparation time: 5 minutes

Cooking Time: 8 hours

Servings: 1

Ingredients:

- 1/2 lb chicken breast, boneless, skinless, cubed
- 1/3 cup celery, chopped
- 1/2 cup carrot, chopped
- 1/2 cup onion, chopped
- 2 oz any kind of mushrooms, sliced
- 1/4 tsp dill weed
- 1/2 tsp Italian seasoning
- 1/4 tsp basil
- 1/4 tsp black pepper
- 1 tomato, diced – limit this

Directions:

1. Place chicken breast cubes into the slow cooker.
2. Add in onion, carrot, Italian seasoning, mushrooms, celery, basil, dill weed, and black pepper. Add in diced tomatoes. Mix well.
3. Seal the lid and cook for 8 hours on low.

4. After the 8-hour cooking cycle, turn off the heat. Adjust seasoning according to your preferred taste.
5. Serve warm.

Nutrition:

Protein: 29.9 g

Potassium: 89.6 mg

Sodium: 56.3 mg

93. Chinese Tempeh Stir Fry

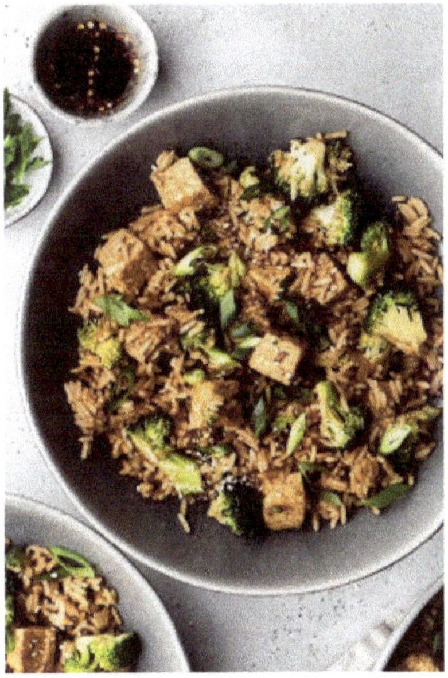

Preparation time: 5 minutes

Cooking time: 15 minutes

Servings: 2

Ingredients:

- 2 oz. sliced tempeh
- 1 cup cooked brown rice
- 1 minced garlic clove
- ½ cup green onions
- 1 tsp. minced fresh ginger
- 1 tbsp. coconut oil

- ½ cup corn

Directions:

1. Preheat the oil in a skillet or wok on a high heat and add the garlic and ginger.
2. Sauté for 1 minute.
3. Now add the tempeh and cook for 5-6 minutes before adding the corn for a further 10 minutes.
4. Now add the green onions and serve over brown rice.

Nutrition:

Calories: 304 Protein: 10g

Carbs: 35g Fat: 4g

Sodium (Na): 91mg

Potassium (K): 121mg

Phosphorus: 222mg

94. Broccoli with Garlic Butter and Almonds

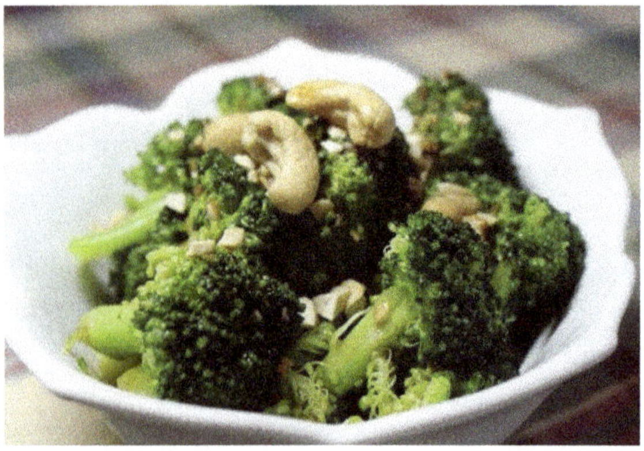

Preparation Time: 10 minutes

Cooking Time: 50 minutes

Servings: 3

Ingredients:

- 1 lb fresh broccoli, cut into bite size pieces
- ¼ cup olive oil
- ½ tablespoon honey
- 1-1/2 tablespoons soy sauce

- ¼ teaspoon ground black pepper
- 2 cloves garlic, minced
- ¼ cup chopped almonds

Directions:

1. Put the broccoli into a large pot with about 1 inch of water in the bottom. Transfer it to strainer and arrange broccoli on a serving platter.
2. Heat the oil in a small skillet over medium heat. Mix in the honey, soy sauce, pepper and garlic.
3. Bring to a boil, then remove from the heat. Mix in the almonds, and pour the sauce over the broccoli. Serve immediately.

Nutrition:

Calories: 177

Sodium: 234mg

Protein: 2.9g

Potassium: 13mg

Phosphorus: 67mg

95. Roasted Garlic Lemon Cauliflower

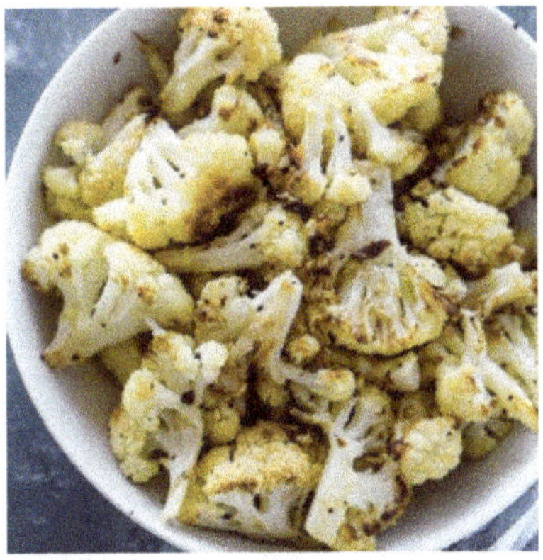

Preparation Time: 10 minutes

Cooking Time: 15 minutes

Servings: 4

Ingredients:

- 2 heads cauliflower, separated into florets

- 2 teaspoons olive oil
- ½ teaspoon ground black pepper
- 1 clove garlic, minced
- ½ teaspoon lemon juice

Directions:

1. Preheat the oven to 400 degrees F.
2. Bake in the preheated oven until florets are tender,for about 15 to 20 minutes.
3. Remove and transfer to a serving platter.

Nutrition:

Calories: 37 Sodium: 27mg

Protein: 1.8g Potassium: 272mg

Phosphorus: 161mg

96. Broccoli with Garlic Sauce

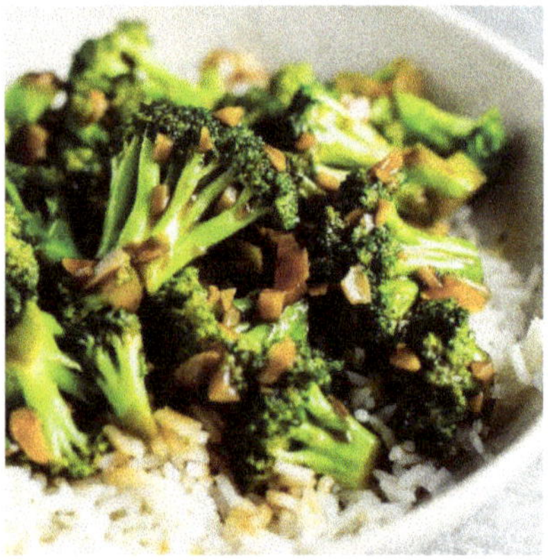

Preparation Time: 10 minutes

Cooking Time: 15 minutes

Servings: 3

Ingredients:

- 2 cups broccoli florets
- 1 garlic cloves
- ½ tablespoon butter
- 2 teaspoons honey

- 1-1/2 tablespoons apple cider vinegar
- 1 tablespoon fresh parsley

Directions:

1. In a large saucepan with steamer rack, steam broccoli over boiling water 8 to 10 minutes or until crisp-tender.
2. Mix in honey, apple cider vinegar and chopped parsley. Return saucepan to heat until sauce is heated.
3. Transfer steamed broccoli to a serving dish.
4. Pour sauce over hot broccoli and toss to coat.

Nutrition

Calories: 41

Sodium: 26mg

Protein: 1.4g

Potassium: 157mg

Phosphorus: 100 mg

97. Parsley Root Veg Stew

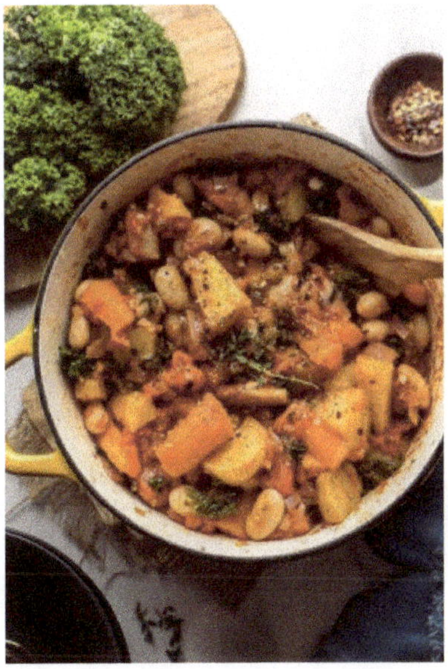

Preparation time: 5 minutes

Cooking time: 35-40 minutes

Servings: 4

Ingredients:

- 2 garlic cloves
- 2 cups white rice
- 1 tsp. ground cumin
- 1 diced onion
- 2 cups water
- 4 peeled and diced turnips
- 1 tsp. cayenne pepper
- ¼ cup chopped fresh parsley
- ½ tsp. ground cinnamon
- 2 tbsps. Olive oil
- 1 tsp. ground ginger
- 2 peeled and diced carrots

Directions:

1. Preheat the oil on a medium high heat before sautéing the onion for 4-5 minutes until soft.
2. Toss in the turnips and cook for 10 minutes or until golden brown.
3. Add the garlic, cumin, ginger, cinnamon, and cayenne pepper, cooking for a further 3 minutes.
4. Add the carrots and stock to the pot and then bring to the boil.
5. Turn the heat down to medium heat, cover and simmer for 20 minutes.
6. Meanwhile add the rice to a pot of water and bring to the boil.
7. Turn down to simmer for 15 minutes.
8. Drain and place the lid on for 5 minutes to steam.
9. Garnish the root vegetable stew with parsley to serve alongside the rice.

Nutrition

Calories: 210

Protein: 4g

Carbs: 32g

Fat: 7g

Sodium (Na): 67mg

Potassium (K): 181mg

Phosphorus: 105mg

98. Lentil Vegan Soup

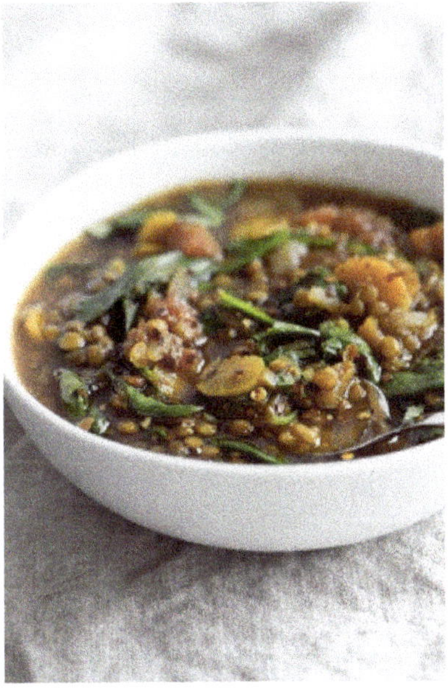

Preparation Time: 10 minutes

Cooking Time: 50 minutes

Servings: 5

Ingredients:

- Olive oil – 2 tablespoons
- Onion (diced) – 1
- Garlic (minced) – 2 cloves
- Carrot (diced) – 1
- Potatoes (diced) – 2
- Tomato (diced) – 1 can (15 ounces)
- Dried lentil – 2 cups
- Vegetable broth – 8 cups
- Bay leaf – 1 - Cumin – ½ teaspoon
- Salt – as per taste
- Pepper – as per taste

Directions:

1. Start by taking a large pot and add in 2 tablespoons of olive oil. Place the pot over medium flame.
2. Once the oil heats through, toss in the onions and cook for 5 minutes.

3. Put in the garlic and cook for another 2 minutes.
4. Now toss in the diced potatoes and carrots. Sauté for about 3 minutes.
5. Add the remaining ingredients like vegetable broth, tomatoes, lentils, cumin and bay leaf. Once it comes to a boil, lower the flame to low and cook for about 40 minutes.take away the the bay leaf and season with pepper and salt. Transfer into a serving bowl. Serve hot!

Nutrition:

Fat: 7g Carbohydrates: 58g

Calories: 364 calories per serving

Protein: 19g

Chapter 16. Poultry Recipes

99. Chicken Fajita Bowls

Preparation Time: 5 minutes

Cooking Time: 15 minutes

Servings: 2

Ingredients:

- Chicken breast - .25 pound
- Olive oil – 1.5 tablespoons
- Onion – 1
- Bell pepper, green – 1
- Bell pepper, red – 1
- Garlic, minced – 4 cloves
- Chili powder - .25 teaspoon
- Cayenne pepper – pinch
- Paprika - .25 teaspoon
- Cumin - .25 teaspoon
- Black pepper, ground - .25 teaspoon
- White rice, cooked – 1.5 cups

Instructions:

1. Combine the chili powder, cayenne pepper, paprika, cumin, and black pepper together to make your fajita seasonings and then set the spices aside.
2. Slice the chicken breast into bite-sized cubes and then place it in a small bowl, massaging it with half of the prepared seasoning mix. Allow it to marinate for fifteen minutes.
3. In a large-sized cooking pan warmed in a stove heat of medium with one tbsp. of the olive oil, cook the bell pepper and onion until soft, about five mins.
4. Add in the chicken and garlic, and continue to cook until the chicken is fully cooked through, reaching an internal Fahrenheit temperature of one-hundred and sixty-five degrees. This should take about ten minutes. Don't forget to stir the chicken occasionally.

5. The skillet should then be removed away from the stove's heat. Serve the vegetables and chicken over the rice.

Nutrition:

Protein Grams: 17

Phosphorus Milligrams: 229

Potassium Milligrams: 510

Sodium Milligrams: 46

Fat Grams: 11

Total Carbohydrates Grams: 47

Net Carbohydrates Grams: 45

100. BlackBerry Chicken Wings

Preparation Time: 35 minutes

Cooking Time: 50 minutes

Serving: 4

Ingredients:

- 3 pounds chicken wings, about 20 pieces
- ½ cup blackberry chipotle jam
- Salt and pepper to taste
- ½ cup of water

Directions:

1. Add water and jam to a bowl and mix well
2. Place chicken wings in a zip bag and add two-thirds of the marinade
3. Season with salt and pepper
4. Let it marinate for 30 minutes
5. Preheat your oven to 400°F
6. Prepare a baking sheet and wire rack, place chicken wings in a wire rack and bake for 15 minutes
7. Brush remaining marinade and bake for 30 minutes more
8. Enjoy!

Nutrition:

Calories: 502

Fat: 39g

Carbohydrates: 01.8g

Protein: 34g

101. Parsley and Chicken Breast

Preparation Time: 10 minutes

Cooking Time: 40 minutes

Serving: 4

Ingredients:

- 1 tablespoon dry parsley
- 1 tablespoon dry basil
- 4 chicken breast halves, boneless and skinless
- ½ teaspoon salt
- ½ teaspoon red pepper flakes, crushed

Directions:

1. Preheat your oven to 350 °F
2. Take ainch baking dish and grease it with cooking spray evenly
3. Sprinkle 1 tablespoon of parsley, 1 teaspoon of basil and spread the mixture over your baking dish
4. Arrange the chicken breast halves over the dish and sprinkle garlic slices on top
5. Use a small mixing bowl and add 1 teaspoon parsley, 1 teaspoon of basil, salt, basil, red pepper and mix well. Pour the mixture over the chicken breast
6. Bake for 25 min.
7. Remove the cover and bake for 15 min.
8. Serve and enjoy!

Nutrition:

Calories: 150

Fat: 4g

Carbohydrates: 4g

Protein: 25g

102. Easy Butternut Chicken

Preparation Time: 15 minutes

Cooking Time: 30 minutes

Serving: 4

Ingredients:

- ½ pound Nitrate free bacon
- 6 chicken thighs, boneless and skinless
- 2-3 cups butternut squash, cubed
- Extra virgin olive oil
- Fresh chopped sage
- Salt and pepper as needed

Directions:

1. Prepare your oven by preheating it to 425 °F
2. Take a large skillet and place it over medium-high heat, add bacon and fry until crispy
3. Take bacon and place it on the side, crumble the bacon
4. Add cubed butternut squash in the bacon grease and Sauté, season with salt and pepper
5. Remove the suash from the pan once tender then transfer to a plate
6. Add coconut oil to the skillet and add chicken thighs, cook for 10 minutes
7. Season with salt and pepper
8. Remove skillet from the stove and transfer to the oven
9. Bake for 12-15 minutes, top with crumbled bacon and sage

Enjoy!

Nutrition:

Calories: 323

Fat: 19g

Carbohydrates: 8g

Protein: 12g

103. Simple Mustard Chicken

Preparation Time: 10 minutes

Cooking Time: 40 minutes

Serving: 4

Ingredients:

- 4 chicken breasts
- ½ cup chicken broth
- 3-4 tablespoons mustard
- 3 tablespoons olive oil
- 1 teaspoon paprika
- 1 teaspoon chili powder
- 1 teaspoon garlic powder

Directions:

1. Take a small bowl and mix mustard, olive oil, paprika, chicken broth, garlic powder, chicken broth, and chili
2. Add chicken breast and marinate for 30 minutes
3. Take a lined baking sheet and arrange the chicken
4. Bake for 35 minutes at 375 °F
5. Serve and enjoy!

Nutrition:

Calories: 531

Fat: 23g

Carbohydrates: 10g

Protein: 64g

–

Chapter 17. Meat Recipes

104. Baked Pork Chops

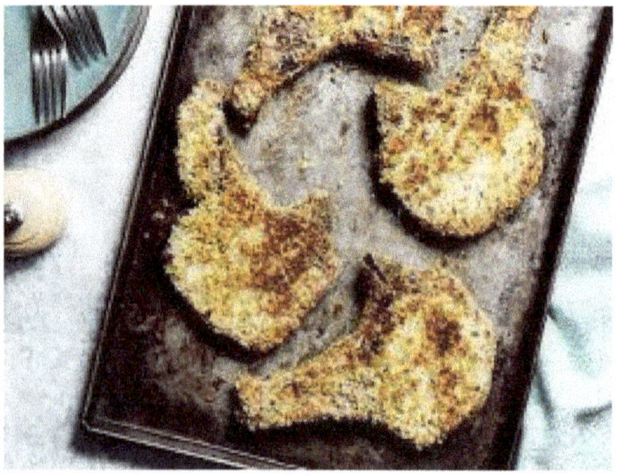

Preparation time: 10 minutes

Cooking time: 40 minutes

Servings: 6

Ingredients:

- 1/2 cup all-purpose flour
- 1 large egg
- 1/4 cup water
- 3/4 cup cornflake crumbs
- 6 (3 1/2 oz) center-cut pork chops
- 2 tbsp unsalted margarine
- 1 tsp paprika

Directions:

1. Preheat oven to 350 degrees F.
2. Mix and spread flour in a shallow plate.
3. Whisk egg with water in another shallow bowl.
4. Spread the cornflakes crumbs in an another plate.
5. Coat the pork with flour then dip in the egg mix and then in the crumbs.
6. Grease a baking sheet and place the chops in it.
7. Sprinkle the paprika on top and bake for 40 minutes.
8. Serve fresh.

Nutrition:

Calories 282.

Protein 23 g.

Carbohydrates 25 g.

Fat 10 g.

Cholesterol 95 mg.

Sodium 263 mg.

Potassium 394 mg.

Phosphorus 203 mg.

Calcium 28 mg.

Fiber 1.4 g.

105. Braised Beef Brisket

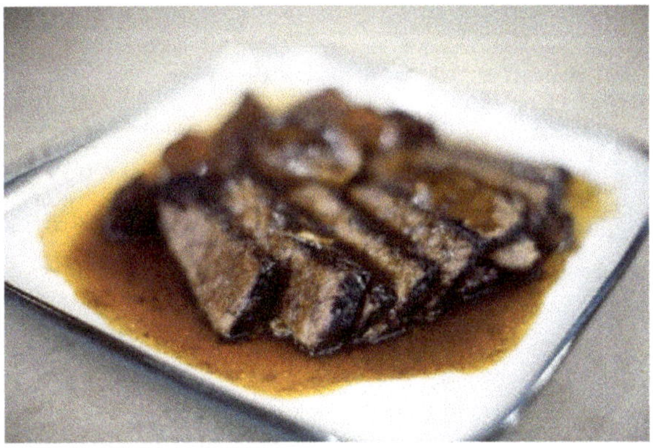

Preparation time: 10 minutes

Cooking time: 1 hour 45 minutes

Servings: 4

Ingredients:

- 1/2 medium onion, sliced
- 1 stalk celery, diced
- 1 medium carrot, diced
- 1 tbsp fresh parsley, chopped
- 2 1/2 lbs beef brisket
- 2 tsp black pepper
- 2 tbsp canola oil

- 3 bay leaves
- 2 cups reduced-sodium beef broth
- 3 cups of water
- 2 tbsp balsamic vinegar

Directions:

1. Preheat oven to 350 degrees F.
2. Remove the fat and season the brisket with black pepper.
3. Warm up the oil in a Dutch oven on medium-high heat.
4. Sear the brisket for 5 minutes and flip to sear for another 5 minutes.
5. Shift this meat to a plate and add carrots, celery, and onion to the pot.
6. Stir fry for 4 minutes.
7. Add bay leaves, parsley and meat over the vegetables.
8. Pour in the water, broth, and balsamic vinegar.
9. Bring it to a boil then cook for 1.5 hours on medium-high heat until meat is tender.
10. Slice the meat and serve with the jus.

Nutrition:

Calories 230.

Protein 29 g.

Carbohydrates 4 g.

Fat 11 g.

Cholesterol 84 mg.

Sodium 178 mg.

Potassium 346 mg.

Phosphorus 193 mg.

Calcium 30 mg.

Fiber 0.8 g.

106. California Pork Chops

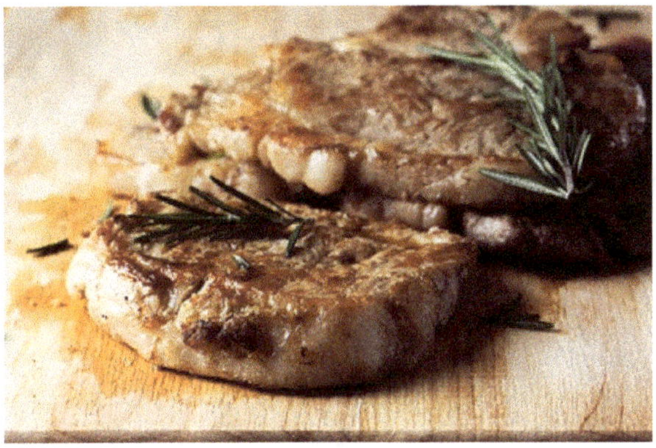

Preparation time: 10 minutes

Cooking time: 10 minutes

Servings: 2

Ingredients:

- 1 tbsp fresh cilantro, chopped
- 1/2 cup chives, chopped
- 2 large green bell peppers, chopped
- 1 lb 1" thick boneless pork chops
- 1 tbsp fresh lime juice
- 2 cups cooked rice
- 1/8 tsp dried oregano leaves
- 1/4 tsp ground black pepper
- 1/4 tsp ground cumin
- 1 tbsp butter
- 1 lime

Directions:

1. Start by seasoning the pork chops with lime juice and cilantro.
2. Place them in a shallow dish.
3. Toss the chives with pepper, cumin, butter, oregano and rice in a bowl.
4. Stuff the bell peppers with this mixture and place them around the pork chops.
5. Cover the chop and bell peppers with a foil sheet and bake them for 10 minutes in the oven at 375 degrees F.

6. Serve warm.

Nutrition:

Calories 265.

Protein 34 g.

Carbohydrates 24 g.

Fat 15 g.

Cholesterol 86 mg.

Sodium 70 mg.

Potassium 564 mg.

Phosphorus 240 mg.

Calcium 22 mg.

Fiber 1.0 g.

107. Beef Chorizo

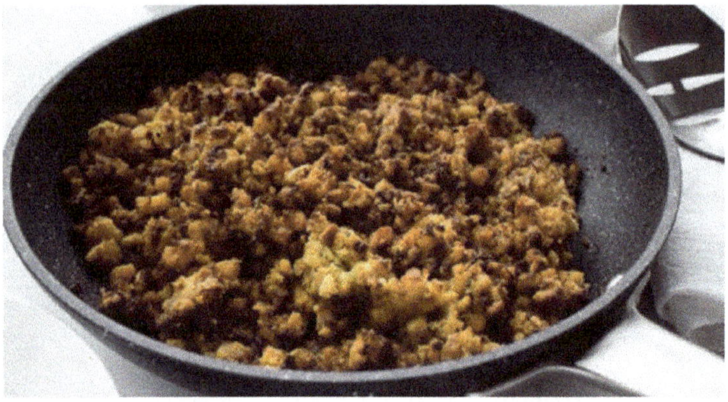

Preparation time: 10 minutes

Cooking time: 10 minutes

Servings: 4

Ingredients:

- 3 garlic cloves, minced
- 1 lb 90% lean ground beef
- 2 tbsp hot chili powder
- 2 tsp red or cayenne pepper
- 1 tsp black pepper

- 1 tsp ground oregano
- 2 tsp white vinegar

Direction:

1. Mix all ingredients together in a bowl thoroughly then spread the mixture in a baking pan.
2. Bake the meat for 10 minutes at 325 degrees F in an oven.
3. Slice and serve in crumbles.

Nutrition:

Calories 72.

Protein 8 g.

Carbohydrates 1 g.

Fat 4 g.

Cholesterol 25 mg.

Sodium 46 mg.

Potassium 174 mg.

Phosphorus 79 mg.

Calcium 14 mg.

Fiber 0.8 g.

108. Onion and Bacon Pork Chops

Preparation Time: 10 minutes

Cooking Time: 45 minutes

Serving: 4

Ingredients:

- 2 onions, peeled and chopped
- 6 bacon slices, chopped
- ½ cup chicken stock
- Salt and pepper to taste
- 4 pork chops

Directions:

1. Preheat up a pan over medium heat and add bacon
2. Stir and cook until crispy
3. Transfer to bowl
4. Bring the pan back to medium heat and add onions, season with salt and pepper
5. Stir and cook for 15 minutes
6. Transfer to the same bowl with bacon
7. Return the pan to heat (medium-high) and add pork chops
8. Season with salt and pepper and brown for 3 minutes
9. Flip and lower heat to medium
10. Cook for 7 minutes more
11. Add stock and stir cook for 2 minutes
12. Return the bacon and onions to the pan and stir cook for 1 minute
13. Serve and enjoy!

Nutrition

Calories: 325

Fat: 18g

Carbohydrates: 6g

Protein: 36g

109. Thai steak salad with herbs and onions

Preparation Time: 10 minutes

Cooking Time: 45 minutes

Serving: 4

Ingredients:

- One flank or rump steak (600 g)
- Salt
- 1 tbsp. peanut oil
- Two red onions
- 1 piece Ginger (20 g)
- One red chili pepper

- One cucumber
- 3 handful Asian herbs (30 g)
- 1 tbsp. rice vinegar
- 3 tbsps. lime juice
- 2 tbsps. Fish sauce
- 1 tsp. honey
- Paprika
- Chili powder
- Pepper
- meat

Directions:

1. Rinse meat, one flank or rump steak, pat dry and salt. Heat the peanut oil and then fry the steak on both sides for 6-8 minutes over high heat. Remove meat from the frying pan and let it rest.
2. Meanwhile, peel onions and ginger. Halve onions and cut into strips. Chop ginger. Cut chili pepper into half lengthwise remove seeds, wash and cut into fine rings. Clean the cucumber, wash, quarter it and slice it. Wash Asian herbs, shake dry and peel off leaves.
3. Add ginger with vinegar, lime juice, fish sauce, honey and 2-3 tablespoons water to a dressing, and mix with paprika, chili powder, salt, and pepper.
4. Slice the meat and arrange with herbs, chili rings, cucumber and onions on a plate and drizzle with the dressing.

Nutrition:

Calories: 390 kcal

Chapter 18. Sauce and Spread Recipes

110. Spicy spread

Preparation Time: 10 minutes

Cooking Time: 45 minutes

Serving: 20

Ingredients:

- 100g butter
- 100g tomato paste
- 200g grated carrots
- 2 cloves of garlic
- 1 onion
- 2 tbsp. Italian herbs (frozen)

Directions:

1. Melt down the butter in a saucepan. Mix it with chop onion and garlic then fry.
2. Also, add the carrots and steam them a little soft so that you can puree them afterward, takes about 5 minutes.
3. Remove from heat and add tomato paste and herbs. Puree and keep in the refrigerator.

Nutrition:

Energy: 44kcal,

Protein: 0g,

Fat: 4g,

Carbohydrates: 1g,

Potassium: 80mg,

Sodium: 14mg,

Calcium: 9mg,

Phosphate: 12mg

111. Bulgur spread

Preparation Time: 10 minutes

Cooking Time: 45 minutes

Serving: 15

Ingredients:

- 100ml vegetable stock
- 50g bulgur
- 100g mushrooms
- 1 tbsp rapeseed oil
- 75g margarine
- Salt, pepper, thyme

Directions:

1. Put the vegetable stock to the boil and let the bulgur soak in it.
2. Cut the mushrooms into small cubes and steam them in the sunflower oil for a minute.
3. Let both cool and puree salt, pepper, and thyme together with margarine.

Nutrition:

Energy: 46kcal,

Protein: 0g,

Fat: 4g,

Carbohydrates: 2g,

Potassium: 29mg,

Phosphate: 17mg

112. Apple and onion lard

Preparation Time: 10 minutes

Cooking Time: 45 minutes

Serving: 2

Ingredients:

- 250g diced onions
- 8 tbsp sunflower oil
- 1 apple
- 100g margarine
- Salt pepper
- 1 teaspoon herbs of Provence

Directions:

1. Steam the onions in the oil until translucent.
2. Peel the apple and grate it finely.
3. Add to the onions and sauté briefly.
4. Season with salt, pepper, and herbs from Provence and let cool.
5. Stir the margarine until creamy and stir in the cooled onion mixture.

Nutrition:

Energy: 52kcal,

Protein: 0g,

Fat: 5g,

Carbohydrates: 1g,

Potassium: 18mg,

Phosphate: 5mg

113. Zucchini spread

Preparation Time: 10 minutes

Cooking Time: 45 minutes

Serving: 2

Ingredients:

- 250 g zucchini
- 60 g double cream cheese with herbs
- 3 tbsp. olive oil
- 1 tbsp. lemon juice

Directions:

1. Wash and clean the zucchini and cut once lengthways.
2. Place the cut side on a greased baking sheet and bake for about 15 minutes at 200 ° C.
3. Remove the zucchini from the oven, let cool down briefly and cut into cubes.
4. Put the zucchini, cheese, oil, juice, and spices in a tall container and puree with the blender.

Nutrition:

Energy: 51kcal,

Protein: 1g,

Fat: 5g,

Carbohydrates: 1g,

Potassium: 50mg,

Sodium: 211mg,

Calcium: 15mg

Chapter 19. Dessert Recipes

114. Dessert Cocktail

Preparation Time: 1 Minutes

Cooking Time: 0 Minute

Servings: 4

Ingredients:

- 1 cup of cranberry juice
- 1 cup of fresh ripe strawberries, washed and hull removed
- 2 tablespoon of lime juice
- ¼ cup of white sugar
- 8 ice cubes

Directions:

1. Toss all ingredients in a blender until smooth and creamy.
2. Pour the liquid into chilled tall glasses and serve cold.

Nutrition:

Calories: 92 kcal

Carbohydrate: 23.5 g

Protein: 0.5 g

Sodium: 3.62 mg

Potassium: 103.78 mg

Phosphorus: 17.86 mg

Dietary Fiber: 0.84 g

Fat: 0.17 g

115. Baked Egg Custard

Preparation Time: 15 minutes

Cooking Time: 30 minutes

Servings: 4

Ingredients:

- 2 medium eggs, at room temperature
- ¼ cup of semi-skimmed milk
- 3 tablespoons of white sugar
- ½ teaspoon of nutmeg
- 1 teaspoon of vanilla extract

Directions:

1. Preheat your oven at 375 F/180C
2. Combine all the ingredients in a bowl then beat with a hand mixer for a few seconds until creamy and uniform.
3. Put the mixture into lightly greased muffin tins.
4. Bake for 25-30 minutes or until the knife, you place inside, comes out clean.

Nutrition:

Calories: 96.56 kcal

Carbohydrate: 10.5 g

Protein: 3.5 g

Sodium: 37.75 mg

Potassium: 58.19 mg

Phosphorus: 58.76 mg

Dietary Fiber: 0.06 g

Fat: 2.91 g

116. Gumdrop Cookies

Preparation Time: 15 minutes

Cooking Time: 12 minutes

Servings: 25

Ingredients:

- ½ cup of spreadable unsalted butter
- 1 medium egg
- 1 cup of brown sugar
- 1 2/3 cups of all-purpose flour, sifted
- ¼ cup of milk
- 1 teaspoon vanilla
- 1 teaspoon of baking powder
- 15 large gumdrops, chopped finely

Directions:

1. Preheat the oven at 400F/195C.
2. Combine the sugar, butter and egg until creamy.
3. Add the milk and vanilla and stir well.
4. Combine the flour with the baking powder in a different bowl. Incorporate to the sugar, butter mixture, and stir.
5. Add the gumdrops and place the mixture in the fridge for half an hour.
6. Drop the dough with tablespoonful into a lightly greased baking or cookie sheet.
7. Bake in the oven for about 10-12 minutes or until golden brown in color.

Nutrition:

Calories: 102.17 kcal

Carbohydrate: 16.5 g

Protein: 0.86 g

Sodium: 23.42 mg

Potassium: 45 mg

Phosphorus: 32.15 mg

Dietary Fiber: 0.13 g

Fat: 4 g

117. Pound Cake with Pineapple

Preparation Time: 10 minutes

Cooking Time: 50 minutes

Servings: 24

Ingredients:

- 3 cups of all-purpose flour, sifted
- 3 cups of sugar
- 1 ½ cups of butter
- 6 whole eggs and 3 egg whites
- 1 teaspoon of vanilla extract
- 1 10. ounce can of pineapple chunks, rinsed and crushed (keep juice aside).

For glaze:

- 1 cup of sugar
- 1 stick of unsalted butter or margarine
- Reserved juice from the pineapple

Directions:

1. Preheat the oven at 350F/180C.
2. Beat the sugar and the butter with a hand mixer until creamy and smooth.
3. Slowly add the eggs (one or two every time) and stir well after pouring each egg.
4. Add the vanilla extract, follow up with the flour and stir well.
5. Add the drained and chopped pineapple.
6. Transfer the mixture into a greased cake tin and bake for 45-50 minutes.
7. In a small saucepan, combine the sugar with the butter and pineapple juice. Stir every few seconds and bring to boil. Cook until you get a creamy to thick glaze consistency.
8. Pour the glaze over the cake while still hot.
9. Let cook for at least 10 seconds and serve.

Nutrition:

Calories: 407.4 kcal

Carbohydrate: 79 g

Protein: 4.25 g

Sodium: 118.97 mg

Potassium: 180.32 mg

Phosphorus: 66.37 mg

Dietary Fiber: 2.25 g

Fat: 16.48 g

118. Apple Crunch Pie

Preparation Time: 10 minutes

Cooking Time: 35 minutes

Servings: 8

Ingredients:

- 4 large tart apples, peeled, seeded and sliced
- ½ cup of white all-purpose flour
- 1/3 cup margarine
- 1 cup of sugar
- ¾ cup of rolled oat flakes
- ½ teaspoon of ground nutmeg

Directions:

1. Preheat the oven to 375F/180C.
2. Place the apples over a lightly greased square pan (around 7 inches).
3. Mix the rest of the ingredients in a medium bowl with and spread the batter over the apples.
4. Bake for about 30-35 minutes, until the top crust has gotten golden brown.
5. Serve hot.

Nutrition:

Calories: 261.9 kcal

Carbohydrate: 47.2 g

Protein: 1.5 g

Sodium: 81 mg

Potassium: 123.74 mg

Phosphorus: 35.27 mg

Dietary Fiber: 2.81 g

Fat: 7.99 g

119. Spiced Peaches

Preparation Time: 5 minutes

Cooking Time: 10 minutes

Servings: 2

Ingredients:

- Canned peaches with juices – 1 cup
- Cornstarch – ½ teaspoon
- Ground cloves – 1 teaspoon
- Ground cinnamon – 1 teaspoon
- Ground nutmeg – 1 teaspoon
- Zest of ½ lemon
- Water – ½ cup

Directions:

1. Drain peaches.
2. Combine cinnamon, cornstarch, nutmeg, ground cloves, and lemon zest in a pan on the stove.
3. Heat on a medium heat and add peaches.
4. Bring to a boil then quickly reduce the heat and simmer for 10 minutes.
5. Serve.

Nutrition:

Calories: 70

Fat: 0g

Carb: 14g

Phosphorus: 23mg

Potassium: 176mg

Sodium: 3mg

120. Tart Apple Granita

Preparation time: 15 minutes, plus 4 hours freezing time

Cooking time: 0

Servings: 4

Ingredients:

- ½ cup granulated sugar
- ½ cup water
- 2 cups unsweetened apple juice
- ¼ cup freshly squeezed lemon juice

Directions:

1. heat the sugar and water.
2. Bring to a boil and then lessen the heat to low and simmer for about 15 minutes or until the liquid has reduced by half.
3. Take away the pan from the heat and pour the liquid into a large shallow metal pan.
4. Let the liquid cool for about 40 minutes and then stir in the apple juice and lemon juice.
5. Place the pan in the freezer.
6. After 1 hour, run a fork through the liquid to break up any ice crystals formed. Scrape down the sides as well.
7. Place the pan back in the freezer and repeat the stirring and scraping every 20 minutes, creating slush.
8. Serve when the mixture is completely frozen and looks like crushed ice, after about 3 hours.

Nutrition:

Calories: 157;

Fat: 0g;

Carbohydrates: 0g;

Phosphorus: 10mg;

Potassium: 141mg;

Sodium: 5mg;

Protein: 0g

121. Lemon-lime Sherbet

Preparation time: 5 minutes, plus 3 hours chilling time

Cooking time: 15 minutes

Servings: 2

Ingredients:

- 2 cups water
- 1 cup granulated sugar
- 3 tablespoons lemon zest, divided
- ½ cup freshly squeezed lemon juice
- Zest of 1 lime
- Juice of 1 lime
- ½ cup heavy (whipping) cream

Directions:

1. Place a large saucepan and add the water, sugar, and 2 tablespoons of the lemon zest.
2. Bring the mixture to a boil and then reduce the heat and simmer for 15 minutes.
3. Transfer the mixture to a large bowl and add the remaining 1 tablespoon lemon zest, the lemon juice, lime zest, and lime juice.
4. Whisk in the heavy cream and transfer the mixture to an ice cream maker.
5. Freeze according to the manufacturer's Directions:.

Nutrition:

Calories: 151;

Fat: 6g;

Carbohydrates: 26g;

Phosphorus: 10mg;

Potassium: 27mg;

Sodium: 6mg;

Protein: 0g

122. Pavlova with Peaches

Preparation time: 30 minutes

Cooking time: 1 hour, plus cooling time

Servings: 3

Ingredients:

- 4 large egg whites, at room temperature
- ½ teaspoon cream of tartar
- 1 cup superfine sugar
- ½ teaspoon pure vanilla extract
- 2 cups drained canned peaches in juice

Directions:

1. Preheat the oven to 225°F.
2. Line a baking sheet with parchment paper; set aside.
3. In a large bowl, beat the egg whites for about 1 minute or until soft peaks form.
4. Beat in the cream of tartar.
5. Add the sugar, 1 tablespoon at a time, until the egg whites are very stiff and glossy. Do not overbeat.
6. Beat in the vanilla.
7. Evenly spoon the meringue onto the baking sheet so that you have 8 rounds.
8. Use the back of the spoon to create an indentation in the middle of each round.
9. Bake the meringues for about 1 hour or until a light brown crust forms.
10. Turn off the oven and let the meringues stand, still in the oven, overnight.
11. Remove the meringues from the sheet and place them on serving plates.
12. Spoon the peaches, dividing evenly, into the centers of the meringues, and serve.
13. Store any unused meringues in a sealed container at room temperature for up to 1 week.

Nutrition:

Calories: 132;

Fat: 0g;

Carbohydrates: 32g;

Phosphorus: 7mg;

Potassium: 95mg;

Sodium: 30mg;

Protein: 2g

123. Tropical Vanilla Snow Cone

Preparation time: 15 minutes, plus freezing time

Cooking time: 0

Servings: 2

Ingredients:

- 1 cup pineapple
- 1 cup frozen strawberries
- 6 tablespoons water
- 2 tablespoons granulated sugar
- 1 tablespoon vanilla extract

Directions:

1. In a large saucepan, mix the peaches, pineapple, strawberries, water, and sugar over medium-high heat and bring to a boil.
2. Lessen the heat to low and simmer the mixture, stirring occasionally, for 15 minutes.
3. Remove from the heat and let the mixture cool completely, for about 1 hour.
4. Stir in the vanilla and transfer the fruit mixture to a food processor or blender.
5. Purée until smooth, and pour the purée into a 9-by-13-inch glass baking dish.
6. Cover and place the dish in the freezer overnight.
7. When the fruit mixture is completely frozen, use a fork to scrape the sorbet until you have flaked flavored ice.
8. Scoop the ice flakes into 4 serving dishes.

Nutrition:

Calories: 92;

Fat: 0g;

Carbohydrates: 22g;

Phosphorus: 17mg;

Potassium: 145mg;

Sodium: 4mg;

Protein: 1g

124. Rhubarb Crumble

Preparation time: 15 minutes

Cooking time: 30 minutes

Servings: 6

Ingredients:

- Unsalted butter, for greasing the baking dish
- 1 cup all-purpose flour
- ½ cup brown sugar
- ½ teaspoon ground cinnamon
- ½ cup unsalted butter, at room temperature
- 1 cup chopped rhubarb
- 2 apples, peeled, cored, and sliced thin
- 2 tablespoons granulated sugar
- 2 tablespoons water

Directions:

1. Preheat the oven to 325°F.
2. In a bowl, mix together the flour, sugar, and cinnamon until well combined.
3. Add the butter and rub the mixture until it resembles coarse crumbs.
4. In a medium saucepan, mix the rhubarb, apple, sugar, and water over medium heat and cook for about 20 minutes or until the rhubarb is soft.
5. Spoon over the fruit mixture into the baking dish and evenly top with the crumble.
6. Bake the crumble for 20 to 30 minutes or until golden brown.

Serve hot.

Nutrition:

Calories: 450;

Fat: 23g;

Carbohydrates: 60g;

Phosphorus: 51mg;

Potassium: 181mg;

Sodium: 10mg;

Protein: 4g

Conclusion

Cooking is a wonderful art. The best part about it is that we can combine ingredients in so many ways, and for so many reasons.

Diabetic? There are recipes for you. High blood pressure? Cooking has you covered. Kidney problems? Get the saucepan and I'll show you some magic.

But you know what makes cooking even more interesting? It's when you bring excitement and fun into your own life. Each meal is prepared with care and love. You end up enjoying the meal because you are getting to enjoy some incredible flavors when you thought you would never be able to. You need to bring the same enjoyment in your life.

I am not a philosopher. But I know that things in life only get harder when our viewpoint on life itself is negative. Think of your health as something you have to take care of and allow it to bring more passion into the way you live. Take steps to live more, smile more, and love more.

At the end of the day, no one can ever claim that they are 100 percent fortunate. Life has a way of showing people tragedies in ways they would never expect. But there is something life cannot do.

It cannot control the way we react.

At this point, you have learned what chronic kidney disease is. You now know what your body is going through and what are the causes. You have also learned how to beware of its symptoms. We have also discussed the benefits of a renal diet. These are just your first steps in working through your diagnosis, or the diagnosis of someone that you love.

Because dealing with Chronic Kidney Disease is a lifestyle change, you will constantly be learning new things and how to help yourself live the best life possible. There are no guarantees that a cure will be found for chronic kidney disease in the near future, but you can start making the first step to avoid dialysis. Catching the disease early on is very crucial, and even if you only fear you may be developing CKD, these tips will help you stop the progression.

Living a kidney-friendly life doesn't mean that you are taking away all of the foods that you love; it just means that you may have to be more diligent in the moderation of your food or fluid intake. When your kidneys are not functioning very well, it can cause strain on the other organs your body depends on to function. That is why early diagnosis is important with chronic kidney disease so that you can be a key player in slowing the progression of the disease by changing your lifestyle.

The resources included in this book are not intended to replace your doctor or a renal dietician, but to give you plenty of options for food choices and seasoning alternatives. You must make sure that you are keeping a journal of the foods you are eating and ones you intend on trying so that your doctor or dietician can help you make an informed decision on whether the diet plan you are trying will work for your stage and severity of kidney disease. Coordination and patience is a key to improving your health.

Life is a conundrum. Its complexities stun us. It surprises and paralyzes us. Its tragedies cripple us. But what life cannot bend, break, change, or destroy is human resilience. You, me, and everyone else on this planet have the same resilience. And that resilience has allowed human beings to face numerous challenges in their lives. Use the same resilience to keep a positive outlook and make healthy changes in your life.

As you live your life experiencing each wonderful dish in this book, know that you are living one more wonderful moment. And sometimes, that is all that is required. One more wonderful moment.

Be more positive. Live with more hope. Eat with more delight.

With much love, I bid you farewell. But I hope you are now thinking of taking a step forward, living your life to the fullest, and enjoying some delicious meals!

Bon appetit.

CPSIA information can be obtained
at www.ICGtesting.com
Printed in the USA
BVHW012028200821
614849BV00003B/60